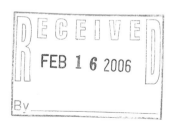

DNA ANALYSIS

FORENSICS:
THE SCIENCE OF CRIME-SOLVING

TITLE LIST

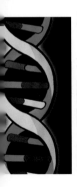

Computer Investigation

Criminal Psychology and Personality Profiling

DNA Analysis

Document Analysis

Entomology and Palynology: Evidence from the Natural World

Explosives and Arson Investigation

Fingerprints, Bite Marks, Ear Prints: Human Signposts

Forensic Anthropology

Forensics in American Culture: Obsessed with Crime

Mark and Trace Analysis

Pathology

Solving Crimes with Physics

DNA ANALYSIS

by William Hunter

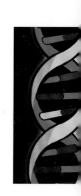

Mason Crest Publishers
Philadelphia

Mason Crest Publishers Inc.
370 Reed Road
Broomall, Pennsylvania 19008
(866) MCP-BOOK (toll free)

First printing
1 2 3 4 5 6 7 8 9 10

Library of Congress Cataloging-in-Publication Data

Hunter, William, 1971–
  DNA analysis / by William Hunter.
      p. cm. — (Forensics, the science of crime-solving)
  Includes index.
  ISBN 1-4222-0026-4   ISBN 1-4222-0025-6 (series)
  1. Forensic genetics. 2. DNA fingerprinting. 3. DNA—
Analysis. 4. Medical jurisprudence. I. Title. II. Series.
  RA1057.5.H86 2006
  614'.1—dc22
                                        2005010082

Produced by Harding House Publishing Service, Inc.
www.hardinghousepages.com
Interior and cover design by MK Bassett-Harvey.
Printed in India.

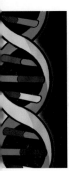

DNA ANALYSIS

Contents

Introduction

By Jay A. Siegel, Ph.D.
Director, Forensic and Investigative Sciences Program
Indiana University, Purdue University, Indianapolis

It seems like every day the news brings forth another story about crime in the United States. Although the crime rate has been slowly decreasing over the past few years (due perhaps in part to the aging of the population), crime continues to be a very serious problem. Increasingly, the stories we read that involve crimes also mention the role that forensic science plays in solving serious crimes. Sensational crimes such as the O. J. Simpson case, or more recently, the Laci Peterson tragedy, provide real examples of the power of forensic science. In recent years there has been an explosion of books, movies, and TV shows devoted to forensic science and crime investigation. The wondrously successful *CSI* TV shows have spawned a major increase in awareness of and interest in forensic science as a tool for solving crimes. *CSI* even has its own syndrome: the "*CSI* Effect," wherein jurors in real cases expect to hear testimony about science such as fingerprints, DNA, and blood spatter because they saw it on TV.

The unprecedented rise in the public's interest in forensic science has fueled demands by students and parents for more educational programs that teach the applications of science to crime. This started in colleges and universities but has filtered down to high schools and middle schools. Even elementary school students now learn how science is used in the criminal justice system. Most educators agree that this developing interest in forensic science is a good thing. It has provided an excellent opportunity to teach students science—and they have fun learning it! Forensic science is an ideal vehicle for teaching science for several reasons. It is truly multidisciplinary;

practically every field of science has forensic applications. Successful forensic scientists must be good problem solvers and critical thinkers. These are critical skills that all students need to develop.

In all of this rush to implement forensic science courses in secondary schools throughout North America, the development of grade-appropriate resources that help guide students and teachers is seriously lacking. There are very few college and high school textbooks and none that are appropriate for younger students. That is why this new series: FORENSICS: THE SCIENCE OF CRIME-SOLVING is so important and so timely. Each book in the series contains a concise, age-appropriate discussion of one or more areas of forensic science.

Students are never too young to begin to learn the principles and applications of science. Forensic science provides an interesting and informative way to introduce scientific concepts in a way that grabs and holds the students' attention. FORENSICS: THE SCIENCE OF CRIME-SOLVING promises to be an important resource in teaching forensic science to students twelve to eighteen years old.

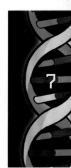

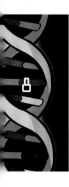

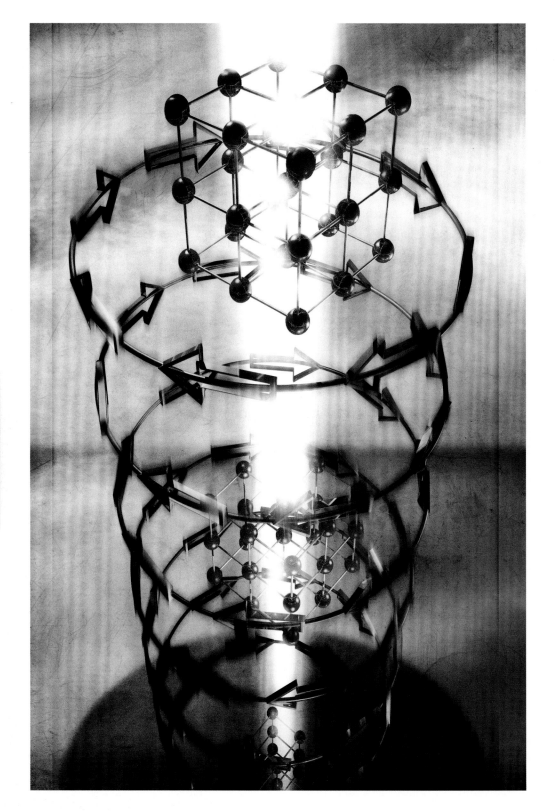

CHAPTER ONE

The Changing Face of Forensic Science

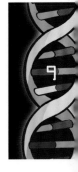

On April 15, 1985, eight-year-old Shandra Whitehead was raped and beaten to death with a rock in her Florida home. The little girl's mother saw a man fleeing from the house, but she did not get a good look at him. Neighbors Chiquita Lowe and Gerald Davis gave somewhat shaky descriptions of a man who had been seen in the neighborhood; one described him as a tall, dark, muscular man wearing an orange T-shirt, while the other remembered him as a droopy-eyed, bearded man. Police artists created composite sketches of the man based on this information.

Two weeks later, the police arrested Frank Lee Smith, whose appearance was similar to the sketch. Smith also had past encounters with the legal system; he had been convicted of murder when he was a teen and served a fifteen-year sentence for that crime. At age thirty-eight, Smith had already spent nearly half his life in prison. Ironically, he was arrested outside Chiquita Lowe's home, where he had gone attempting to sell a television set. Lowe went on to serve as the *prosecution's* prime witness.

Frank Lee Smith went on trial for Shandra's murder based on two reports that a man who looked like him was in the neighborhood at the time the crime was committed and on the mother's identification of him as the man she had seen leaving her house, though she had initially been able to provide little description. The prosecution presented no physical evidence linking Smith to the crime, even though this type of crime is usually accompanied by significant physical evidence. Smith was convicted and sentenced to death under Florida law.

Chiquita Lowe later admitted she did not feel Smith was the man she had seen but had felt pressured by her family and the police to identify him as Shandra's attacker. Her testimony was critical for the conviction.

Trial watchers in Florida began studying the case several years after the sentencing. Jeff Walsh, a private investigator, showed Chiquita Lowe a picture of a man known to have a history of crimes like Shandra's rape and murder. Lowe immediately recognized Eddie Lee Mosley as the man she had seen the night of the murder. Mosley had been suspected of several sex crimes in the region, yet for some reason the police did not investigate whether he had been involved, even after Chiquita Lowe *recanted* her testimony.

The change in Chiquita Lowe's testimony sparked years of legal battles in Florida courts. For ten years, lawyers fought to free Frank Lee Smith. Although they were unable to get his conviction reversed, they did successfully keep him from being executed. Finally, in 1998, when advanced DNA testing became admissible as evidence in trials, his lawyers submitted their first request to check Smith's DNA against the evidence collected at the scene of the crime. State prosecutors resisted this, fighting to avoid the testing of the evidence. Eventually the state did test the evidence, revealing that the DNA found at the scene of the crime in fact matched Eddie Lee Mosley's and not Frank Lee Smith's DNA.

Smith spent fourteen long years on death row for a crime he did not commit. Finally, in December of 2000, he was

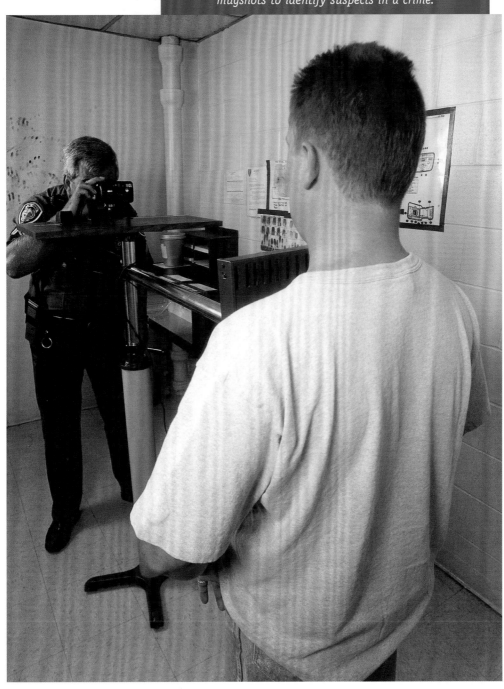

Today, investigators still rely on fingerprints and mugshots to identify suspects in a crime.

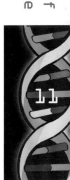

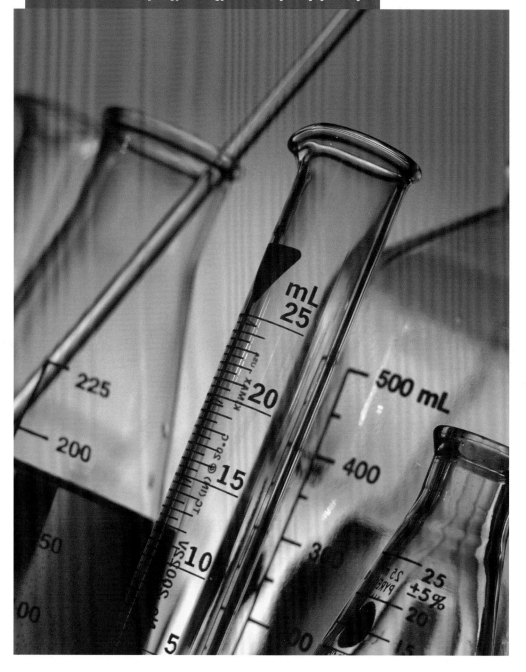

Forensic scientists are usually highly specialized in one or two areas like anthropology, biology, chemistry, or psychiatry.

officially cleared of all charges. However, it was too late for him to enjoy his freedom. While the state had resisted the DNA testing, Smith died of cancer in prison. He was cleared only after his death.

A BRIEF INTRODUCTION TO THE FORENSIC SCIENCES

A flake of skin . . . a strand of hair . . . a fleck of saliva . . . a drop of blood. Everywhere we go, we leave behind bits of ourselves that are as unique to us as our fingerprints. Scientists today can look into our very cells to tell us apart. The average, law-abiding citizen is probably not that concerned about this, but a small segment of our population cares very deeply about the record they leave behind.

There have always been individuals who feel they are above the law, who do not care what effect their actions have on other people around them. Crimes are committed every day around the world. Over time, people have developed a number of ways to find and prove that someone has committed a crime. The field of science that deals with crimes and the interaction between law and science has come to be known as forensic science. The earliest recorded use of forensic science techniques dates back to seventh-century China, where vendors used inks to imprint a bill of debt with the fingerprint of their customers as proof of the debt.

Awareness of forensic science has grown among the public, but for years scientist crime fighters worked silently in the background, helping investigators solve crimes while getting little recognition. Oddly, the increased attention can probably be attributed to entertainment. Sir Arthur Conan Doyle's famous character, Sherlock Holmes, was one of the first well-known literary figures using forensic science. Many years later, the comic strip character Dick Tracy had a wide following. In more recent times, the amazingly popular television show *CSI: Crime Scene Investigation* has been credited with helping to

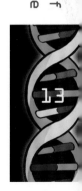

make forensic science one of the most rapidly growing career paths a student can choose in college.

CSI portrays the forensic scientist as a jack-of-all-trades, but in reality forensic scientists are typically highly specialized in one or two areas of forensics. What viewers see on *CSI* has been dressed up for television. Most forensic scientists do not go from crime scene to crime scene examining evidence, grilling witnesses, and helping the police make arrests. Still, the job can be exciting and fulfilling for the people who choose forensics as a career. How many people can honestly say they helped put a murderer behind bars?

Forensic science is an umbrella term used to describe the whole group of specialized careers used to help solve crimes. Within forensic science, there are a number of different areas, each with their own requirements and applications. Forensic science laboratories often include anthropologists, biologists, chemists, computer specialists, dental specialists, physicists, and psychiatrists. The types of scientists found in each laboratory depends on the funding the lab receives and the sorts of crimes it is normally called on to help solve.

Each specialist within a forensic laboratory deals with a relatively narrow area of evidence. Chemists might be asked to examine traces of gasoline found at the scene of a fire thought to have been started by an arsonist. Computer specialists can study the information on a computer found at a crime scene to look for clues in the files or documents that have been saved on the machine. Physicists are skilled at using their knowledge of angles and the behavior of matter to figure out where a bullet might have come from, or how a particular blood spatter pattern might have been created during the commission of a crime.

Crime scene evidence that contains any kind of biological tissue, including blood, skin, saliva, semen, hairs, or sweat, is within the realm of forensic biologists. The majority of the work that forensic biologists do at present involves DNA evidence. DNA evidence, however, is not the only type of bodily evidence important in crime investigation. Long before the discovery of DNA, a basic bodily fluid—blood—was used to help solve crimes.

A BRIEF HISTORY OF THE USE OF BLOOD IN CRIMINAL CASES

DNA profiling is a relative newcomer on the forensic science scene. The technology that allows a skilled technician to examine a sample of blood or other body tissue and provide valuable

Some forensic scientists specialize in computers, tracking evidence by searching files saved on a computer found at the crime scene.

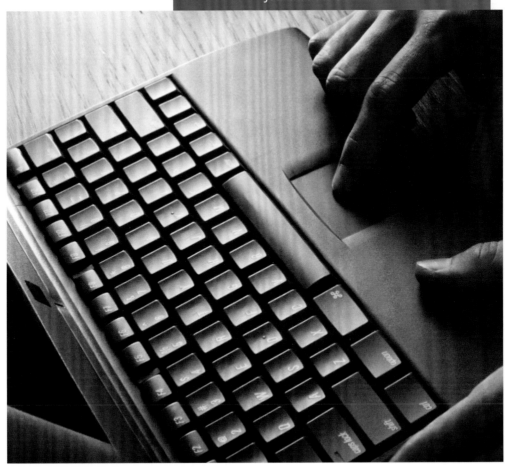

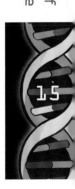

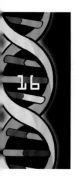

At a crime scene, an investigator has many tools she can use to find tiny amounts of blood that could otherwise go unnoticed. A creative investigator might find traces of blood underneath the tiles of a floor by pouring water on the tiles and watching to see where it flows. She might dig deeper into her forensic bag of tricks and use luminol spray to find the tiny spots of blood. When sprayed on an area thought to contain blood, luminol reacts to give off a faint blue light. In a very dark room, bloodstains stand out like the stars against the night sky. As the amount of blood present increases, so does the brightness of the glow caused by the reaction.

insights as to who it came from is new enough that it is still greeted with a great deal of skepticism by lawyers and judges around the world.

No crime scene investigator in the world, however, will deny that the presence of blood is critically important evidence at a crime scene. Blood may well be the single most important type of evidence commonly found.

Most people have about ten pints of blood flowing throughout their bodies, and it is under relatively high pressure. When a person is wounded during a crime, blood can spray or leak into the most unlikely places. A trained

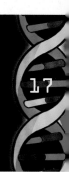

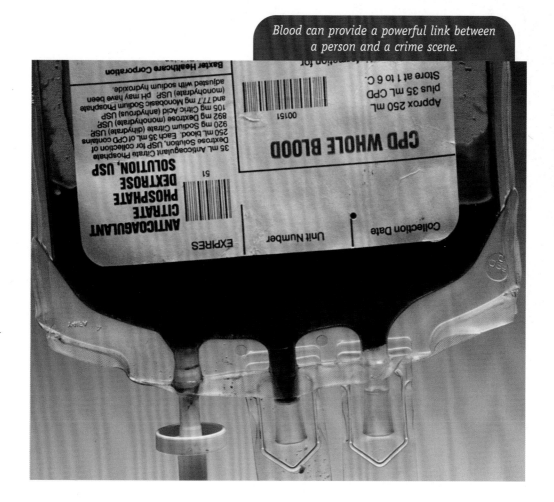

Blood can provide a powerful link between a person and a crime scene.

crime-scene investigator has the tools and experience to know how to find it. Blood can provide a powerful link between a person and a crime scene. It can be pretty tough for a person to explain the presence of his blood at the scene of a murder or the victim's blood on his clothing or in his car.

Blood is actually a mixture of many cells, each with a specific function necessary for life. All blood has two major components: plasma and cells. Plasma is the liquid in which the blood cells float. It contains proteins, nutrients for other cell types, salts, and cellular waste products. Most of the fluid that flows out when a person is cut is plasma. The cells of blood—which include red blood cells, white blood cells, and platelets—each have a specific purpose. Red blood cells, which give blood its color, carry oxygen throughout the body and bring carbon dioxide to the lungs to be exhaled. Mature red blood cells do not have nuclei, so they contain no nuclear DNA. Platelets are responsible for blood clotting when a person is cut. Platelets also lack such DNA. White blood cells are part of the immune system, responding to infections and illnesses. Every white blood cell has a nucleus, so they are a valuable source of DNA for evidence.

Table 1: Blood Types

Type O+	33% (One out of three people)
Type A+	33% (One out of three people)
Type B+	8.3% (One out of twelve people)
Type O–	6.7% (One out of fifteen people)
Type A–	6.3% (One out of sixteen people)
Type AB+	3.4% (One out of twenty-nine people)
Type B–	1.5% (One out of sixty-seven people)
Type AB–	0.6% (One out of one hundred sixteen seven people)

Scientists have known since 1875 that blood can be separated into distinct types. However, it was not until 1901 that a scientist named Karl Landsteiner developed a system for identifying each one. Landsteiner's work laid the foundation for what we now call the ABO system of blood typing, which is still used today. The ABO typing system provided the basis for the development of modern-day crime-solving techniques and served as a springboard for the use of DNA profiling to help put criminals behind bars.

The ABO blood type of a person depends on the types of proteins she has in her blood. There are four major blood types: A, B, AB, and O. Every person in the world has one of these

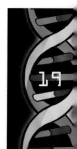

Unlike white blood cells, red blood cells have no nucleus and therefore do not contain nucleic DNA.

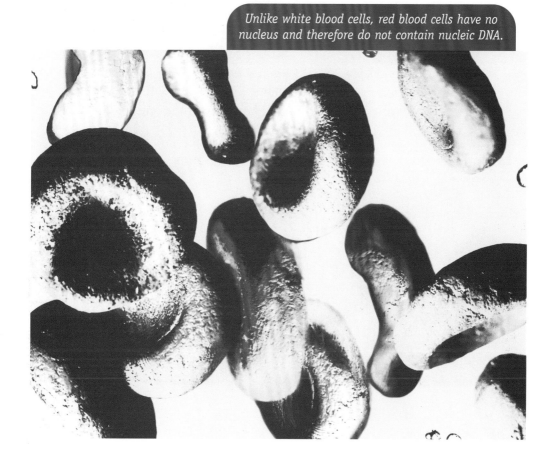

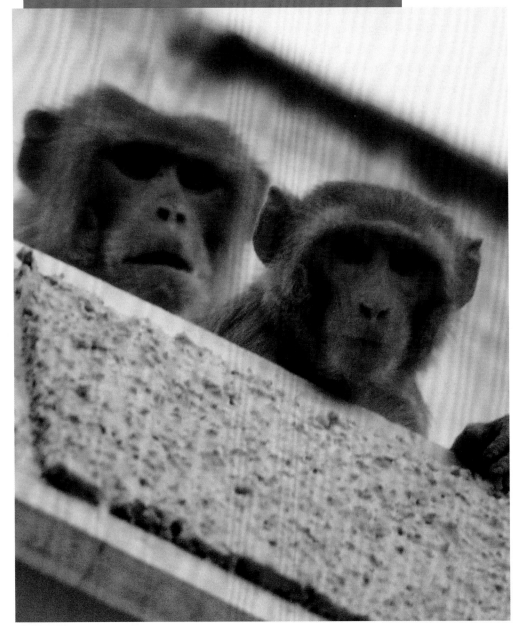

The Rhesus factor, a protein sometimes found in human blood, was named after Rhesus monkeys, who have the protein in common.

four blood types, a useful way to narrow the number of suspects from which a sample of blood could have come.

Landsteiner is also credited with the discovery of another protein, which he called the *Rhesus* factor (rH). The name comes from the fact that he found the same protein in the blood of *Rhesus* monkeys. People are either rH positive (+) if they have the protein in their blood or rH negative (–) if they do not. Nearly 85 percent of all people are rH positive. The use of rH factor allows forensic scientists to further reduce the number of people from which a particular sample might have come.

Blood-typing has been used in criminal investigation for many years. The main problem with using blood type as evidence is that it is not specific enough to be considered strong evidence. Blood types alone are not enough to convict a person of a crime. Table 1 contains data about the numbers of people worldwide of each major blood type. Notice that no blood type could be used to narrow down the number of possible matches to less than 1 in 167. Considering that there are billions of people in the world, there is far too high a chance that the sample could have come from more than one person for this sort of evidence to be useful as the sole means of identification.

In others words, finding type A+ blood at the scene of a crime cannot be used to positively identify a person, because 33 percent of all people in the world have the same blood type. Obviously, however, blood-typing can rule out a person, if their blood is a different type than that found at the scene. Blood type remains useful as evidence, but it alone is not nearly enough to ensure a conviction.

The development of DNA technology has changed the field of forensic science, providing evidence that scientists, lawyers, and judges did not even dream about in the old days.

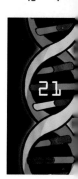

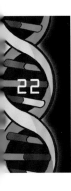

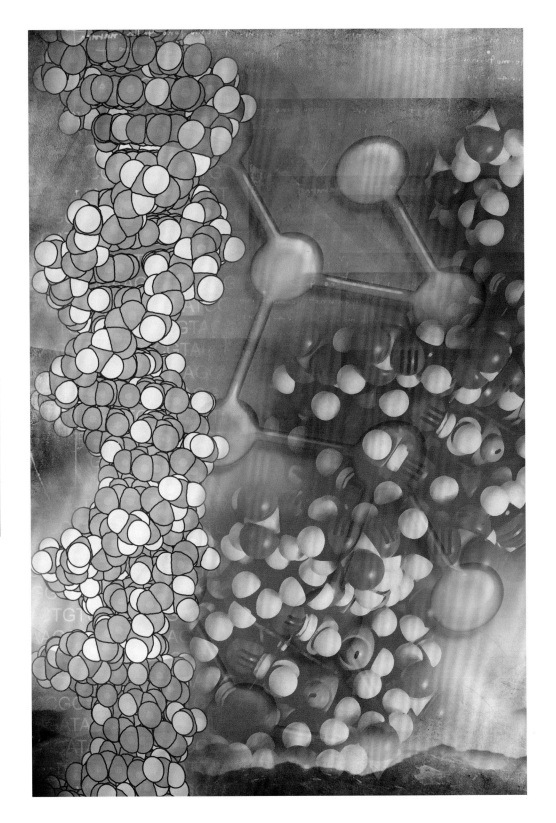

CHAPTER TWO

Introducing . . . DNA!

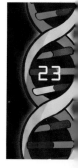

In 1981, a fisherman named Clyde Charles was walking out of a bar when the police arrested him for rape. Earlier that night, a police officer had seen him hitchhiking in the same area where a nurse was mugged and raped after her car broke down, and he matched the description given by the victim.

Charles was tried and convicted by a jury based on the victim's identification, including her testimony that the rapist called himself "Clyde." In addition, Charles had two hairs on his clothing when he was arrested that experts testified were similar to the victim's, though they were unable to say for sure if the hairs were hers.

Nearly ten years later, Charles began a letter-writing campaign to convince authorities to use the DNA technology that had become widely available in the intervening years to compare his DNA to samples found at the scene of the crime. Charles's case was taken up by the Innocence Project, an organization that advocates for convicted criminals trying to establish their innocence. Pressure from the Innocence Project, combined with media coverage by the PBS show *Frontline*, eventually resulted in the reexamination of the evidence using modern technology.

Luckily, the samples had been properly preserved, and scientists were able to use DNA fingerprinting to analyze the evidence. The DNA testing revealed that Clyde could not have been the man to leave the samples. Instead, the evidence turned out to have been left by a man Clyde knew quite well: his brother Marlo, who had allowed Clyde to be tried and convicted and then to serve more than fifteen years in prison for a crime Marlo knew for certain he had not committed. Clyde was released from prison in 1999.

WELCOME TO THE WORLD OF DNA

The discovery of DNA in 1953 and the subsequent development of techniques for analyzing it may be the single most important development in forensic science in many, many years. In 1984, Dr. Alec Jeffreys discovered that each person on this earth has unique DNA, except identical twins. The use of a special technique known as DNA fingerprinting quite rapidly became a powerful tool for *molecular biologists* and *geneticists*. The legal community, however, has always been far less eager to adopt new ideas. Dr. Jeffreys' work opened the door for exploration into the use of DNA technologies in crime fighting, but it took many years for the courts to accept the new evidence in trials. New developments in the field of molecular biology have made DNA evidence very powerful in the courtroom, perhaps more powerful than any other type of evidence. Few types of evidence can link a person to a crime scene with as much certainty as DNA.

Most people have heard of DNA, whether in science class or in a book or movie, but the average person might not know much about what it is. DNA is an acronym for deoxyribonucleic acid. It is present in nearly every cell of a person's body and has an important role to play in determining exactly what those cells are like. It works as an instruction manual for the

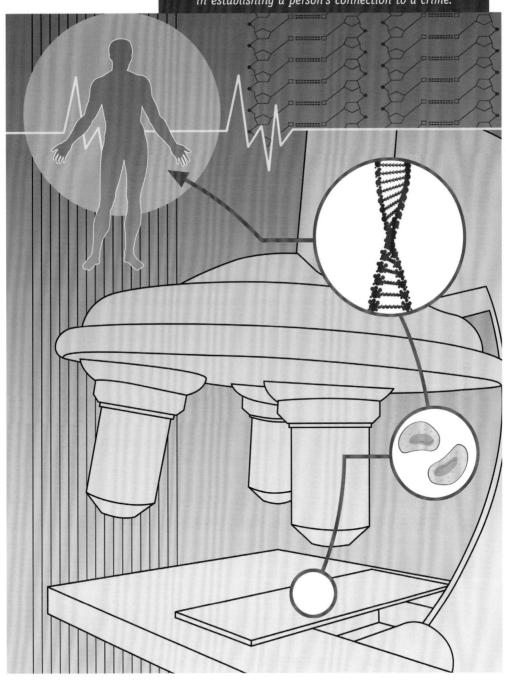

Because every person (except identical twins) has unique DNA, DNA fingerprinting can play an integral role in establishing a person's connection to a crime.

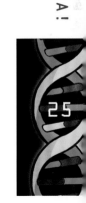

cells in the body, telling each cell what job to do, whether it is a blood cell, a muscle cell, or any other type of cell. Special techniques in molecular biology allow forensic technicians to extract the DNA and make it a useful investigative tool. A single cell can provide enough DNA for a skilled scientist to link a person to a crime scene.

DNA has a molecular structure called a double helix, which looks something like a spiral staircase. Each individual strand is made up of over three billion parts, called bases, arranged in a continuous chain that twists around the other strand. There are four bases that make up the majority of all DNA: adenine, thymine, guanine, and cytosine. One strand of DNA is complementary to the other in a double helix; adenine always pairs with thymine, while guanine always pairs with cytosine. This is the basis of how DNA can be replicated.

The arrangement of the bases determines a person's genetic makeup. A person inherits one strand of DNA from each of his parents, which explains why traits can pass from generation to generation. The DNA in one cell is exactly the same as the DNA in every other cell in a person's body. It is extremely rare for any two people to have identical DNA. In fact, the only people who do share the same DNA are identical twins because they come from the splitting of one fertilized egg.

The chances of unrelated people having the same DNA are very low (so low that it is almost impossible), making DNA a useful molecule for crime investigation. It is true, however, that the majority of DNA is the same in everyone. In fact, as much as 99 percent of all DNA is identical from person to person. However, considering that there are more than three billion bases in a strand of DNA, that one percent of difference can add up to a huge number of different bases from person to person. One percent of three billion is thirty million, more than enough to differentiate between two people.

Crime-scene investigators are trained to find DNA sources—anything that could harbor a few human cells. Objects such as cigarette butts, skin under the fingernails of a

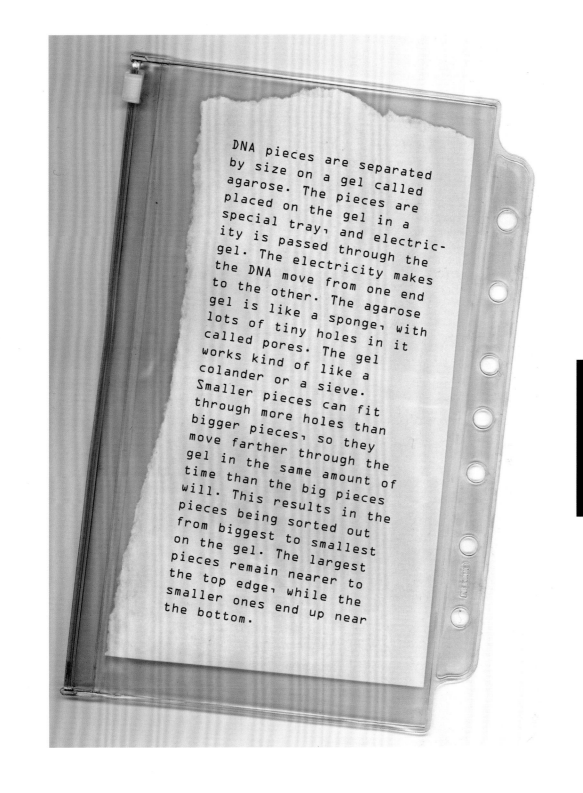

DNA pieces are separated by size on a gel called agarose. The pieces are placed on the gel in a special tray, and electricity is passed through the gel. The electricity makes the DNA move from one end to the other. The agarose gel is like a sponge, with lots of tiny holes in it called pores. The gel works kind of like a colander or a sieve. Smaller pieces can fit through more holes than bigger pieces, so they move farther through the gel in the same amount of time than the big pieces will. This results in the pieces being sorted out from biggest to smallest on the gel. The largest pieces remain nearer to the top edge, while the smaller ones end up near the bottom.

DNA can be extracted from tiny samples of hair, skin, blood, semen, and saliva.

victim, pieces of clothing, and even doorknobs have proven to hold enough cells from which to gather DNA evidence. A tiny bit of skin can have more than enough cells to prove valuable to the skillful forensic biologist in her laboratory. Bloodstains are also a very good source of DNA. Once a DNA source is found, the scientist can remove the DNA from the cells and begin the process of examining it.

DNA FINGERPRINTING

The genetic analysis technique called DNA fingerprinting has several steps. First, scientists have to cut the DNA into small pieces. Obviously, DNA is already too tiny to cut using scissors or knives, so scientists use special chemicals called enzymes to break the DNA into pieces. Enzymes are special proteins that have very specific functions. Restriction enzymes can find specific DNA sequences and break the DNA apart at that sequence. These enzymes are derived from bacteria that use them to break up the DNA of any organism they might invade. Next, the scientist separates the pieces by size using a process involving a special gel.

Once the gel has finished running and the DNA fragments are fully sorted according to their sizes, the technician transfers the fragments to a strong but thin membrane, then places the membrane on top of an X-ray film and exposes the membrane to X-rays, creating a sort of "photograph" of the pattern of DNA fragments. This process allows each gel to be compared to other samples and to be stored for a long period of time. The gels are not very strong and are liable to rip if moved, making the membrane transfer an important part of the process. The fragment sizes will vary for different people, allowing a fingerprint of the DNA to be developed. When a forensic scientist compares the fingerprint of a known sample, taken from each suspect in front of a reliable witness, to that found at a crime scene, the fingerprint can be used as evidence that a person was present at the scene at some time. If two samples match perfectly, chances are they came from the same person. DNA

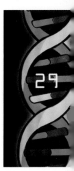

fingerprinting is very time consuming and expensive, requiring many hours of a technician's time to complete one sample analysis.

The strands of DNA that are used during DNA fingerprinting are called variable number tandem repeats (VNTRs). These sections of DNA can be hundreds of base pairs long and will repeat along the strand of DNA any number of times (leading to the use of the term "variable number").

DNA AS EVIDENCE

If DNA evidence is going to be used in court, it needs to be reliable. Jurors need assurances that the sample could not have come from someone other than the accused before a sample can be admitted as evidence. An expert would need to testify about the odds that the sample came from someone other than the accused. Luckily, DNA fingerprinting can produce some fairly compelling evidence when properly established by an expert.

Two different but similar standards govern what scientific evidence is admissible in court, depending on where the case is heard. Some areas use the standard from the 1923 case, *Frye v. United States*, which held that the court can accept expert testimony when it is "sufficiently established" and "generally accept[ed]" in the scientific community and is based on "well recognized scientific principle and discovery." This means that new science has to be pretty thoroughly accepted before it is allowed in court. Other areas use the standard from a more recent case, *Daubert v. Merrell Dow Pharmaceutical, Inc.* This case allows evidence to be admitted if it has been subjected to *peer review*, is *standardized*, has a known *error rate*, and has achieved widespread acceptance. Under either standard, DNA evidence is generally considered admissible in courts, unless there is something in a particular case that makes it less reliable than usual.

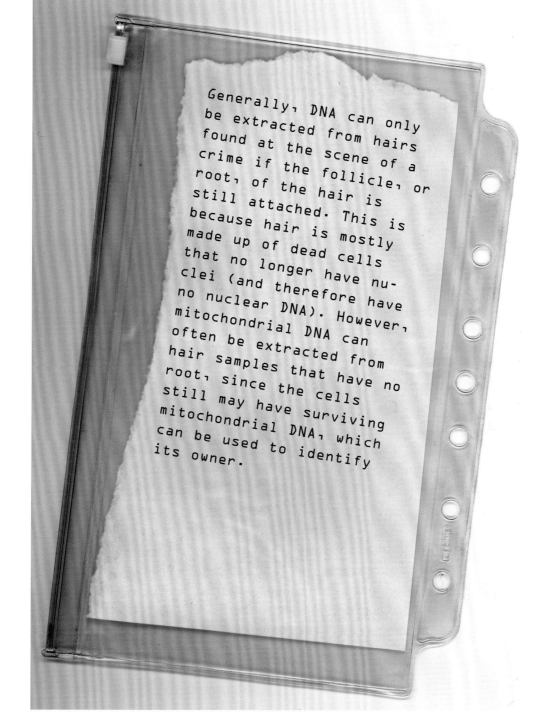

Generally, DNA can only be extracted from hairs found at the scene of a crime if the follicle, or root, of the hair is still attached. This is because hair is mostly made up of dead cells that no longer have nuclei (and therefore have no nuclear DNA). However, mitochondrial DNA can often be extracted from hair samples that have no root, since the cells still may have surviving mitochondrial DNA, which can be used to identify its owner.

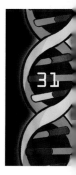

MITOCHONDRIAL DNA: ANOTHER TOOL IN THE TOOLBOX

All the DNA we have discussed thus far, and most DNA used in a criminal investigation, is found in the nucleus of the cell, called nuclear DNA, coming from the twenty-three pairs of chromosomes that are in the nuclei of our cells. This is probably what most people think about when they think of DNA. However, DNA is also found in a cell's mitochondria, small *organelles* that produce energy for the cell. Unlike nuclear DNA, which is inherited from both parents, mitochondrial DNA stays exactly the same from generation to generation (except in the very unlikely case of a mutation) and is passed only from mother to child. This means your mitochondrial DNA is exactly like your mother's, your grandmother's, your great-grandmother's, and so on. Mitochondrial DNA is sometimes available in situations where nuclear DNA is not.

Each *mitochondrion* has a copy of the mitochondrial DNA in it, and each cell in the body has hundreds or thousands of mitochondria, meaning that there are hundreds or thousands of copies of the mitochondrial DNA in each cell. Although each nucleus has a copy of the nuclear DNA, each cell has only one nucleus and therefore only one copy. The increased number of copies of mitochondrial DNA results in an increased chance that some will have survived in situations that might damage DNA, such as when a body has been badly burnt.

Although mitochondrial DNA testing has some advantages over the nuclear DNA testing that is usually done, it is not the standard in criminal cases. For starters, while no two people have the same nuclear DNA (unless they are identical twins), everyone in the same family line has the same mitochondrial DNA. That does not mean mitochondrial DNA has no value, because it can certainly increase the likelihood that the sample found at the crime scene belongs to the suspect, but it cannot establish it with the same degree of certainty as nuclear DNA testing can. Of course, this disadvantage can also serve as an advantage, since a DNA sample taken from a suspect's brother

CASE STUDY: THE BOSTON STRANGLER

The city of Boston was terrorized during the early sixties by a series of rapes and murders during which women were strangled in their apartment with an article of clothing. The papers began calling the perpetrator the Boston Strangler, though police were not sure that the same person committed all the crimes. While in jail on unrelated serial sexual assault charges, Albert DeSalvo confessed the strangulations to another inmate. Many people believed that DeSalvo was mentally ill and had not committed the crimes, some believed he was mentally ill and had committed the crimes, while others thought he was mentally competent and indeed the Boston Strangler. The prosecution was unable to establish enough evidence that DeSalvo had committed the murders. DeSalvo pleaded guilty to the unrelated crimes, and no one was ever charged in the Boston Strangler killings, though many felt the true perpetrator was in prison. DeSalvo was murdered by another inmate in 1973.

More than thirty-five years after the last Boston Strangler murder, the final victim, Mary Sullivan, was exhumed from her grave. A semen stain on her body was tested for DNA. Although no nuclear DNA had survived the intervening years, scientists did find mitochondrial DNA. The investigators used Albert DeSalvo's brother Richard's blood to get a sample of mitochondrial DNA, which would be identical to Albert DeSalvo's. Instead of confirming that DeSalvo was Sullivan's killer, as many expected, the tests revealed that the semen did not belong to DeSalvo, making it far less likely he had committed the crime.

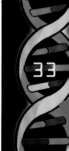
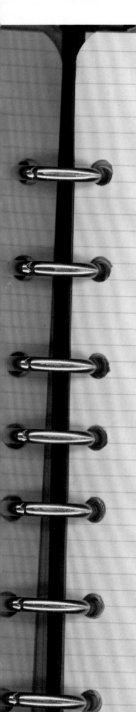

(or sister, mother, grandmother, or even the child of a female suspect) will serve just as well as a sample from the suspect himself, since his mitochondrial DNA will be identical to anyone who is from the same maternal line.

In addition, mitochondrial DNA testing is much more time consuming and expensive than nuclear DNA testing. Most laboratories are not set up to do these tests at this time. The FBI laboratory does mitochondrial DNA testing, but will only do it in FBI cases and under limited circumstances.

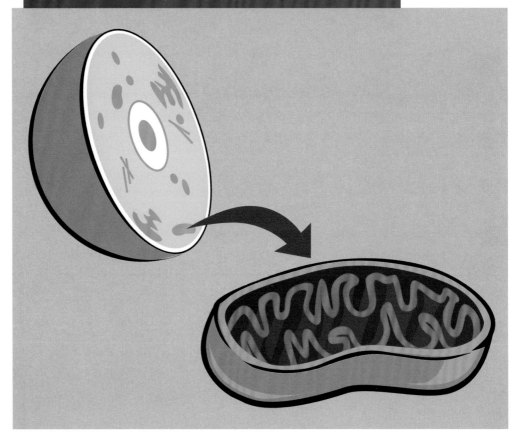

Mitochondria, found in every cell, contain genetic information that stays constant throughout the generations. Mitochondrial DNA can provide familial links.

Mitochondrial DNA looks very different from nuclear DNA. Rather than one long strand of base pairs, mitochondrial DNA is made up of a loop of base pairs. This loop has thirty-seven genes on it, all of which are used in making energy, the job of a mitochondrion. Scientists have found two sections of mitochondrial DNA, the hypervariable regions, that are very different from person to person. In order to analyze them, a polymerase chain reaction (PCR) is used to create many copies of the region, and then the base pairs are *sequenced*. This process takes a long time and is quite complex, and the results are less certain than with nuclear DNA testing.

As a result of the expense and increased handling time of DNA fingerprinting, the difficulties and costs of working with mitochondrial DNA, and advances in technology, a new and much more powerful technique was developed: DNA profiling.

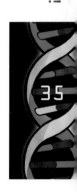

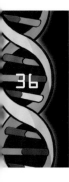

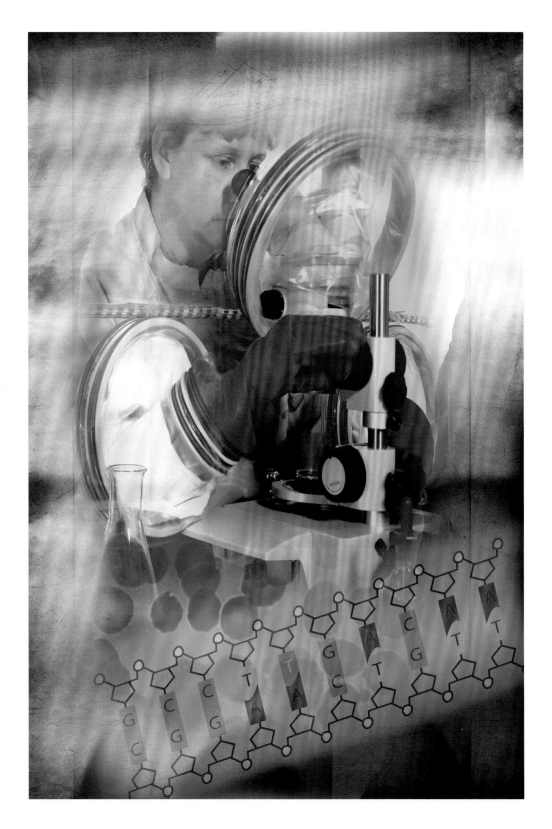

CHAPTER THREE

DNA Profiling: A Beginner's Guide

In 1995, Ricky McGinn was convicted and sentenced to death for the rape and murder of his twelve-year-old step-daughter, whose bloodied body had been discovered in a ditch. The trial went relatively quickly, with McGinn maintaining his innocence throughout the proceedings. The evidence was piled up against him, but he refused to admit he had done the crime. Even after spending six years on Texas death row, McGinn continued to claim he was innocent. He began to focus on trying to stay alive, looking for a way to get off death row.

Under Texas law, the murder alone would not have been enough to condemn McGinn to death; the rape made the crime a capital felony, triggering the death penalty. As a result, McGinn turned his attention to disproving that he was the rapist. Evidence from the rape examination, including semen and a single pubic hair, could be tested using new DNA techniques that would provide a more reliable picture of what really happened that day.

McGinn hired a few high-profile attorneys to spearhead his attempt to be cleared of the rape charge based on DNA evidence. He began telling the Texas media he had been framed.

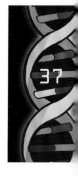

McGinn insisted that the police had planted the evidence against him because they needed to get a conviction. George W. Bush, the governor of the state at the time, ordered the evidence tested with the new techniques, just to be sure.

McGinn continued to assure people he was innocent and the tests would prove it. He was wrong. The pubic hair yielded DNA that exactly matched that of Ricky McGinn. The police had the right man after all. McGinn's execution was rescheduled, and he died of a lethal injection on September 27, 2000. He had apparently hoped that the test would be inaccurate, but it was not.

AN INTRODUCTION TO DNA PROFILING

In light of the difficulties and limitations of using DNA finger-printing or mitochondrial DNA sequencing as evidence, researchers needed to discover a new, faster, and more accurate

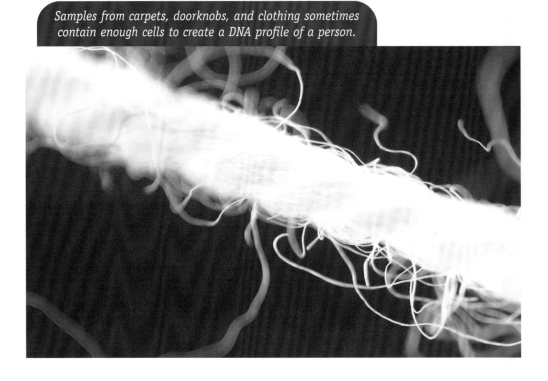

Samples from carpets, doorknobs, and clothing sometimes contain enough cells to create a DNA profile of a person.

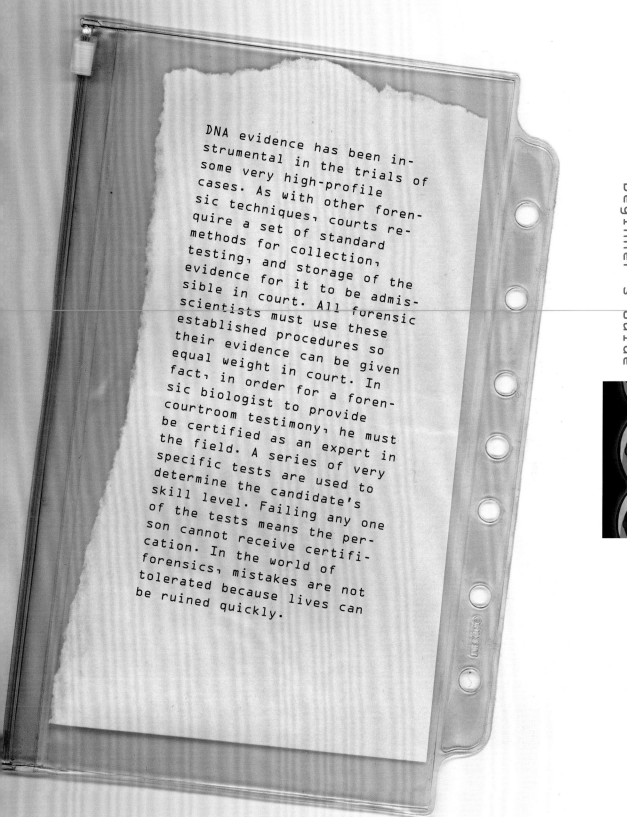

DNA evidence has been instrumental in the trials of some very high-profile cases. As with other forensic techniques, courts require a set of standard methods for collection, testing, and storage of the evidence for it to be admissible in court. All forensic scientists must use these established procedures so their evidence can be given equal weight in court. In fact, in order for a forensic biologist to provide courtroom testimony, he must be certified as an expert in the field. A series of very specific tests are used to determine the candidate's skill level. Failing any one of the tests means the person cannot receive certification. In the world of forensics, mistakes are not tolerated because lives can be ruined quickly.

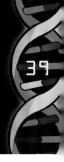

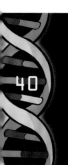

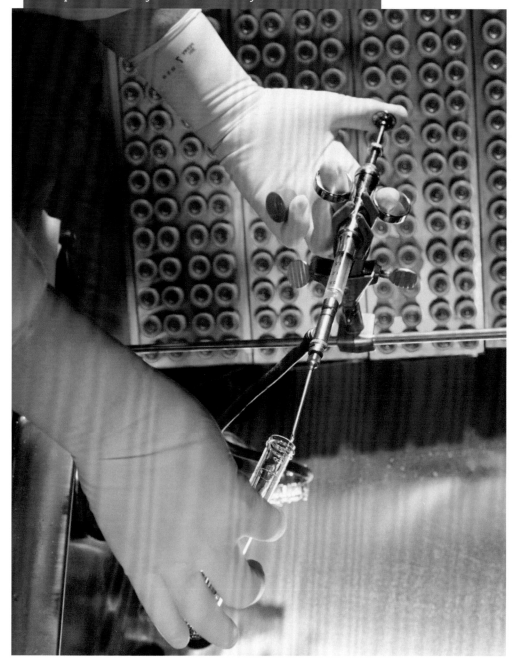

Most forensic laboratories have huge freezers full of stored samples in case they are needed even after a case is closed.

method of processing DNA samples from crime scenes and other forensically important sources.

A method of DNA profiling using very short segments of DNA came onto the forensic scene in the late 1990s as new technology became more and more widespread. The ability to use smaller and smaller samples was of obvious value to forensic scientists, who pushed for the acceptance and use of the new techniques in crime fighting. Crime scenes often yield very little evidence, and any method that can help make even the smallest shred of evidence more useful is critical to their work.

HOW DNA PROFILES ARE MADE

Scientists follow a series of steps to make a DNA profile. The first step is obviously finding the DNA source, either at the crime scene or from a sample taken from a suspect to be compared to that found at the scene of the crime. Luckily, a very small amount of tissue is all that is needed. A single hair found at the crime scene is often enough, if the root of the hair is still attached. Blood is full of DNA, and if a blood spot is big enough to be visible, there are hundreds of thousands of cells available.

The next step, the actual DNA extraction process—when the DNA is taken out of the cells—is perhaps the simplest part of the procedure. The tissue or blood is placed in a small tube with several very carefully measured chemicals. One of these is a *buffer* solution that keeps the DNA from falling apart, which it will do if the buffer is left out. The other substances are designed to break down the cells and release the DNA into the buffer. Normally, a scientist can do this part of the process in less than an hour. Then she will usually divide the samples into several identical units so that some can be saved in a freezer in case they are needed later. Most forensic laboratories have huge freezers full of samples because they must be kept for many years after the investigation in case they are needed again.

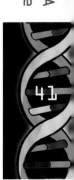

Once the DNA extraction is complete, the scientist can start the next step of the process. She uses a UV spectrophotometer to determine how much DNA she extracted. Light rays of a specific wavelength are passed through the sample. (Like water, light travels in waves, and wavelength is the distance between the peak of one wave and the peak of the next.) High-energy wavelengths, like UV rays (the part of sunlight that causes a sunburn), have waves that are closer together than lower-energy wavelengths, like the part of sunlight that you can see. Different types of molecules absorb different wavelengths of light, so the UV spectrophotometer sends out rays that are absorbed by the DNA. A sample with more DNA in it will absorb more of this light. Scientists can do some simple mathematical calculations to determine how much DNA is present based on the amount of light that is absorbed. (See chapter 6 for more information about the tools used to extract DNA.)

THE POLYMERASE CHAIN REACTION

One single extraction does not usually produce enough DNA for analysis, so scientists use the polymerase chain reaction (PCR) process to amplify, or increase, the amount of DNA available. This process is pretty complicated and requires special equipment, but it has made it possible to get useful DNA from much smaller amounts of evidence collected at a crime scene.

The scientist follows several steps to complete the PCR process. He combines the sample containing the DNA with a special enzyme called DNA polymerase that produces copies of DNA when the conditions are right. These conditions include mixing adenine, thymine, guanine, and cytosine (the raw materials of DNA), and a few other chemicals with the DNA sample. The scientist also adds a set of specially designed *primers*, which are little bits of DNA that provide instructions about where to start and where to stop copying the long strand that is in the sample.

The primers are a necessary part of the reaction because it is not yet possible to copy a whole DNA molecule in one reaction. In general, PCR amplifications must be kept under one thousand bases long, because the accuracy of the copying process decreases greatly beyond this point. No technology exists at this time that allows scientists to simply copy the entire length of a DNA molecule. Therefore, the amplification must be done in short segments. By carefully selecting the primers, scientists can amplify sections of DNA that they know are likely to be different from one person to the next.

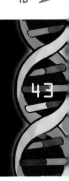

Scientists use a UV spectrophotometer to pass light through a sample to determine how much DNA is present.

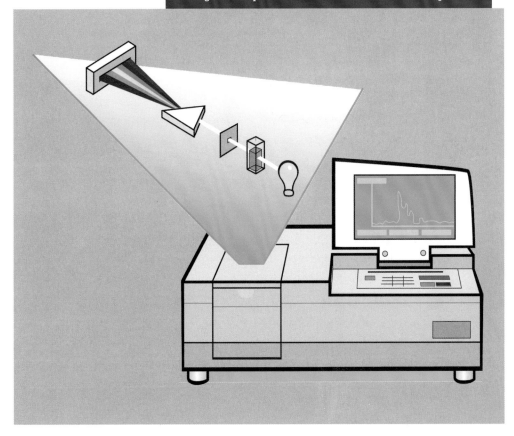

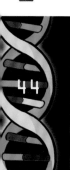
The other important condition involves carefully changing the temperature of the solution. By doing this, the technician can create copies of parts of the DNA in the sample. The solution is placed in a special machine called a thermocycler that controls the temperature of the reaction. When the temperature is raised to approximately 203 degrees Fahrenheit (about 95 degrees Celsius), the paired strands of DNA in the solution untwist from one another, kind of like unzipping a zipper, a process called denaturation. Once the strands are denatured, the temperature is reduced to allow the primers to *anneal*, or attach, to the now separate strands. After the primers attach

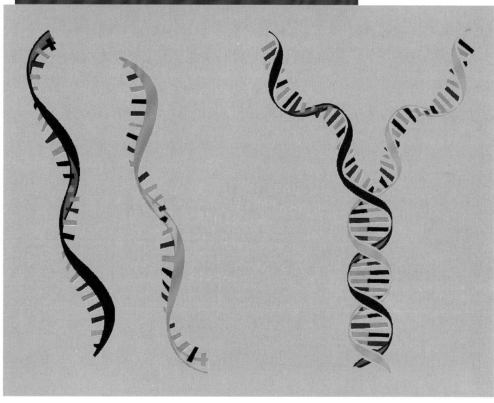

To increase the amount of DNA in a sample, the entwined strands of the double helix must first be "unzipped" so that new base pairs may attach to them.

The short sections of DNA
called STRs are stable
enough that they have
even survived for liter-
ally thousands of years
in the tombs of ancient
Egypt. Scientists from
Brigham Young University
extracted DNA from hun-
dreds of Egyptian mum-
mies, commoners and
pharaohs alike. The STRs,
which will show similari-
ties among closely re-
lated individuals, al-
lowed the scientists to
draw conclusions about
family relationships
among mummies, even es-
tablishing things like
brother-sister marriages
in the royal line.

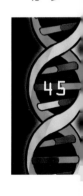

to the single strand, the polymerase attaches to the primer and creates new strands of the DNA by moving along the existing strand and attaching complementary bases in a chain during the extension step of the reaction. The polymerase moves from one primer to the other and then detaches. The short strands produced by the polymerase then link up with each other and form very short double helixes.

A single cycle in the thermocycler goes through each of these steps once. Typically the reaction is run for twenty to thirty cycles. For each double helix in the starting solution, two copies of the desired parts can be produced in each cycle. For example, if the reaction started with just one double helix of DNA, at the end of the first cycle there would be two double helixes. At the end of a second cycle there would be four double helixes in the solution. Each successive cycle doubles the number of double helixes in the solution, eventually giving the biologist enough DNA to examine. If the forensic biologist started with just two DNA molecules, twenty cycles of PCR would create over two million exact copies of the sequence desired.

SHORT TANDEM REPEATS

The newest technique for forensic analysis of DNA is called the polymerase chain reaction-short tandem repeat (PCR-STR) method. Scientists have been able to identify short sections of DNA that tend to be different from one person to the next. Through PCR amplification of several of those DNA sections, biologists can determine with a high degree of certainty whether the sample from the crime scene matches samples taken from any suspect. STRs are those segments of DNA that are made up of between three and seven repeated base sequences (the sequence ATAT, for example: adenine, thymine, adenine, thymine). Each STR is repeated many times, but the actual number of repeats varies from person to person, which is how they can be used to tell the difference between two people. For example, consider the commonly used STR known as TH01. In

A very important factor in
determining whether a DNA
test is useful for crime-
solving purposes is its
specificity. Evidence that
leaves little doubt that it
could have only come from one
person is highly specific.
With every DNA test, there is
a small chance that a sample
might have come from someone
other than the person in
question. However, when a
test is highly specific,
those chances are extremely
small. For example, a typical
DNA fingerprint carries a one
in three hundred million
chance that it could have
come from more than one person on the planet. An STR
test using just ten of the
thirteen core loci often has
less than one in three trillion chance of having come
from two different people.
Obviously, STRs are far more
specific than DNA finger-
printing.

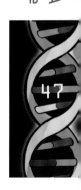

one person, the sequence might look something like this: -AATG-AATG-AATG-AATG-AATG-. In another person, the sequence might be: -AATG-AATG-AATG-. The sensitive equipment used to analyze the samples easily picks out the smaller section of repeats, and the graph of the differences is a nice visual display to show in court.

One great benefit of STR analysis is how quickly the results can be obtained. A skilled lab technician can usually produce a profile in about five hours from start to finish. STR primers can all be combined in one neat reaction, reducing the cost and amount of handling during sample processing. Many of the big biotechnology companies now produce STR kits that further simplify the whole process, reducing the amount of sample handling to a bare minimum while increasing accuracy. The less often people touch a sample, the less likely it is that someone will make a mistake with it.

The short length of the STR fragments means they are much more stable than DNA fingerprint fragments. DNA of longer length is more likely to break apart under normal conditions, meaning that STR evidence can be recovered from badly decayed bodies in situations where DNA fingerprinting would be impossible.

The human *genome* contains literally hundreds of STR sequences. Because of the way they are inherited and how much they vary from person to person, the more STRs a forensic scientist can attribute to a sample, the smaller the chance becomes of that sample matching more than one person. In forensic laboratories, a technique known as multiplexing is used to streamline the process. More than one STR can be amplified in a single PCR step, saving valuable time for the forensic biologist working the case. Multiplexing has been made even easier by the development of commercial kits containing all of the chemicals and primers needed to *amplify* the entire set of STRs; these are commonly used by most crime labs in the country.

Segments of DNA containing certain sequences of
base pairs vary from person to person.

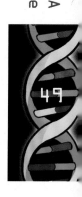

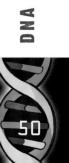

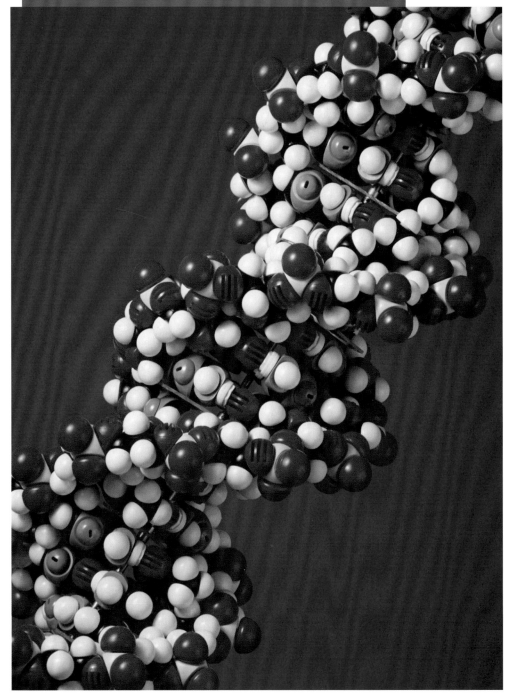

A model shows the many components found in a portion of DNA.

The FBI recommends investigative analysis of thirteen different STRs that can be found on different parts of a person's DNA. These are called the core *loci*, and they are named either according to where they can be found or what their function is. This is important because most parts of DNA are the same from person to person. The core loci were selected for use in identifying individuals because they are found in nearly every person in the world, yet are extremely variable from person to person. Therefore, they can be used to match samples with such certainty that it is virtually impossible to argue that a sample of DNA could have come from more than one person.

STR analysis continues with the injection of the amplified DNA into a computerized machine that passes a focused beam of light through the sample in much the same way that is used to determine the amount of DNA present. The machine then displays a graph that shows the number of repeats for each STR. Few people in the world (other than identical twins) have the exact same number of repeats in all thirteen core loci, allowing a forensic scientist to determine with great certainty whether a sample from an unknown individual matches that of a suspect. Nothing in science is ever considered absolutely true, but STR analysis gets pretty close to it.

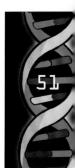

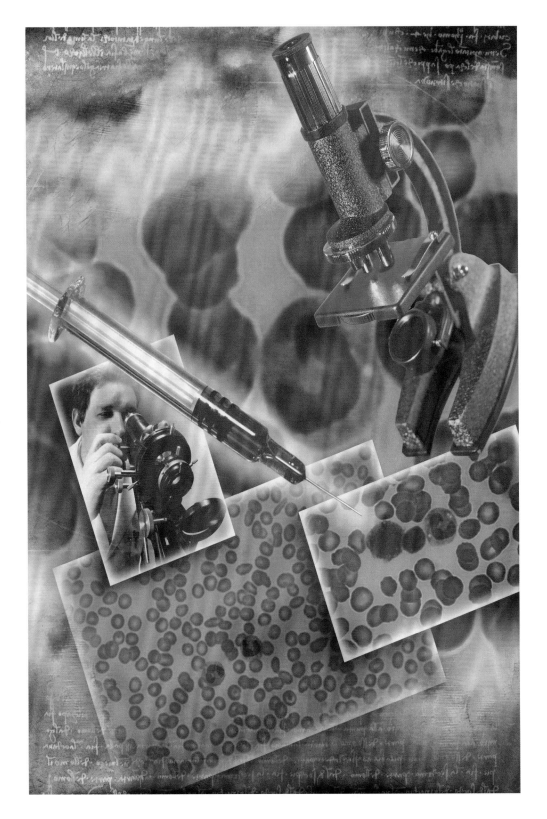

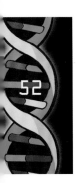

CHAPTER FOUR

Evidence and Accuracy

In May of 1995, the world was watching as popular former NFL star and actor O. J. Simpson's DNA went on trial. The trial hinged on the blood that was found at the scene of the crime, a bloodied sock and glove found at Simpson's Los Angeles house, and a small spot of blood found inside the defendant's car. If the prosecution could prove to the jury that the blood evidence indicated Simpson was present at the scene of the crime, and that the blood found on the sock at the foot of his bed belonged to his dead former wife or her friend (who was also murdered at the crime scene), Simpson would have a very difficult time maintaining his innocence, especially when paired with the high-profile car chase the world had watched following the murders.

Simpson hired a team of eleven of the best lawyers in the country to fight the charges against him. He had twenty-five more lawyers working from offices to find ways to discredit the evidence and introduce doubt to the jury. The case might well be the most publicized trial in the history of the United States. It ran over nine month's time, and cost the state of California and Simpson over $20,000,000. The trial stirred up a media

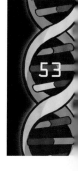

frenzy, with constant TV coverage of every aspect. A circus owner might have been proud to call it an attraction under his big top.

In spite of the blood evidence, the prosecution's case had some weaknesses. The prosecution had no eyewitness that could place O. J. at the scene of the crime. No actual evidence found at the scene of the crime (except for the blood) could show that he had been there that night. In fact, Simpson was not even in Los Angeles when the police came to question him about the murder; he was in Chicago. The man living in a bungalow on Simpson's estate, Kato Kaelin, had mentioned he had seen Simpson leave his house at about 10:45 P.M. for a flight. Kaelin also said he had heard three loud thumps coming from behind his bungalow shortly before then.

After hearing from Kaelin about the sounds, detectives searched around the bungalow and discovered the bloody glove that appeared to be a right-handed match for one found at the scene of the crime. Wisely, they left the glove alone until crime-scene specialists arrived to collect it. The police officers also found what appeared to be blood spots inside a vehicle belonging to Simpson, parked on the street nearby. After obtaining a search warrant, officers came across the bloody sock at the foot of the bed, inside the master bedroom.

As the trial wore on, it became apparent that the prosecution would have to show that the blood found on the glove and sock linked Simpson to the crime. The prosecution had put together a long list of evidence against Simpson, but due to some very skillful work by the defense team, the focus became the blood evidence and the bloody glove.

The world watched while O. J. tried on the glove. It did not fit! This easily understandable visual demonstration (and attorney Johnny Cochran's "If it doesn't fit, you must acquit") trumped the scientific evidence. In spite of testimony from a prosecution expert witness that the blood found at the scene of the crime had a 1 in 170 million chance of having come from someone other than O. J. Simpson, and the blood on the glove and sock almost certainly came from Nicole Brown Simpson, the defense was able to shed doubt on the validity of the evidence. DNA evidence had been thrust into the spotlight, but it would be years before it was fully accepted in courts.

STRIVING FOR ACCURACY

DNA profiling can be a very powerful tool for solving all sorts of criminal and civil cases, but what makes it so good? STR analysis is a very new technique in forensic science, but like all other forms of evidence, rules apply for collection, testing, and storage. A high level of accuracy and a low risk of error is one requirement of the legal community, and using the thirteen core loci allows scientists to meet these requirements. With the

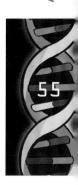

A leather glove similar to the one that played a major role in the O. J. Simpson trial

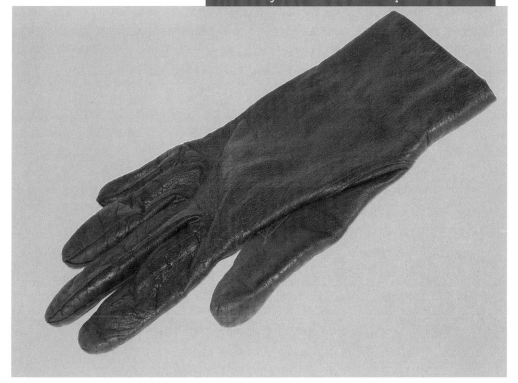

development of better equipment and techniques, the entire process has been made extremely rapid and accurate. The level of specificity of a properly done STR profile is truly amazing.

Over the years, the legal community has become more and more accepting of STRs and DNA evidence in general, largely because of the many success stories. Of course, there will always be a chance that a mistake could be made, but with standardization of the technique, and the usage of the same thirteen loci in every laboratory in the country, it is more likely that errors could occur in evidence collection than in processing. Commercial kits are available now that make it more likely for STR analysis to be accepted in court because of the ability to exactly re-create the results in an independent retesting of the samples.

DNA profiling has gained acceptance within the legal community over the years because it provides highly accurate results with a low probability of error.

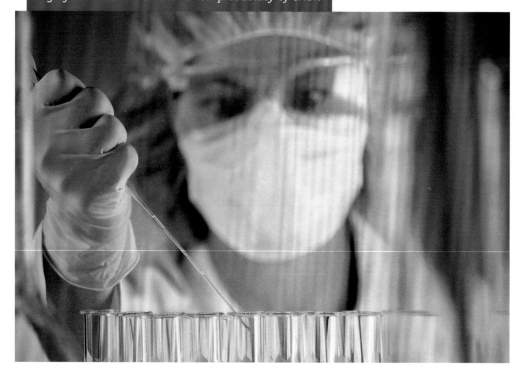

When the forensic biologist runs a sample of unknown DNA through the STR process, he always runs a control sequence alongside it. The use of control sequences, which are extremely pure DNA samples that have been carefully selected to serve as an indicator of whether the amplification was successful, helps provide additional assurances that the data is accurate. Since the scientist knows exactly what to expect from the control sequence, he can assume the reaction worked properly if the control sequence profile matches the results from the last time he used it.

HOW ACCURATE IS IT?

The main reason DNA profiling is so useful is that it provides an amazing level of certainty that a particular pattern of STR types could not likely have come from more than one person. Scientists can spout statistics that seem unbelievable when linking one DNA sample to a particular individual using this technology. Often, the chance of two people having the same STR pattern is less than one in three trillion. To understand how staggeringly small the chances are that there are two people with the same STR pattern, consider that the current population of the world is around 6.5 billion. The odds against an

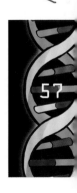

Table 2: STR Frequencies

Example of a table of STR frequencies for a typical white male. Locus refers to the STR core loci. Genotype indicates how many repeats of each loci the individual has in the profile (two numbers indicate he is heterozygous for that particular loci). Frequency is the percentage of white males that have the same genotype for that particular loci. The odds of any other person having the exact same DNA profile for these thirteen loci are approximately 1 in 7.7 quadrillion! (1 in 7,700,000,000,000,000). The final column, AMEL, reveals whether the suspect was male or female.

Locus	D3S1358	VWA	FGA	D8S1179	D21S11	D18S51	D5S818
Genotype	15, 18	16, 16	19, 24	12, 13	29, 31	12, 13	11, 13
Frequency	8.2%	4.4%	1.7%	9.9%	2.3%	4.3%	13%

Locus	D13S317	D7S820	D16S539	THO1	TPOX	CSF1PO	AMEL
Genotype	11, 11	10, 10	11, 11	9, 9.3	8, 8	11, 11	X Y
Frequency	1.2%	6.3%	9.5%	9.6%	3.52%	7.2%	(Male)

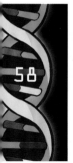

The National Center for Biotechnology Information (NCBI) maintains a massive database of DNA sequence information that is freely available to the general public. The sequences are largely contributed by researchers at universities, who use the sequence data to help them answer questions about what purpose a particular section of DNA has in human development. Visit www.ncbi.nlm.nih.gov/ for more information about the NCBI database, or to browse the sequence files.

STR pattern being duplicated are more than the total population of the whole planet!

The scientific community shows little doubt that STR profiles are a valuable and accurate source of evidence. However, the same cannot be said of the legal community. Debate has raged since the very first use of DNA as evidence, and many people believe that it is likely to continue for years to come. In many cases, jurors have simply ignored DNA evidence, partly because it is hard for people to really understand the tiny chance that a DNA sample could have come from more than one person. People have a hard time wrapping their minds around

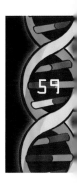

Figure 1: DNA chart

1

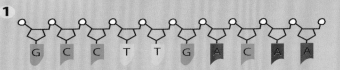

DNA is made up of four bases, **A**denine, **T**hymine, **C**ytosine, and **G**uanine, which are linked in a strand.

2

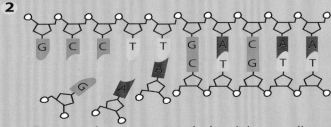

Two complementary strands then join according to basic pairing rules: the **A**s of one strand pair with the **T**s of another strand, and the **C**s pair with the **G**s.

3

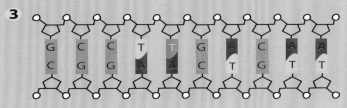

The result is a double-stranded DNA molecule.

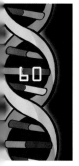

The Hardy-Weinberg Principle may be one of the most powerful theories in biological science, but like most other theories, it operates on some basic assumptions. At its heart is the assumption of random mating. In most populations, the individuals do select mates randomly. There are a few cases where breeding has become nonrandom, however. Domestic dogs, for example, are often bred with others having traits the owner wants in the puppies. This is directed breeding, and the Hardy-Weinberg Principle will not apply. The formula cannot be used to calculate the puppies' allele frequencies.

one in three trillion, because we do not usually deal with numbers that huge.

USING THE EVIDENCE

With all types of evidence, there are very strict rules for specificity and accuracy. When the rules are not met, evidence is usually not used or is even thrown out of court. In addition, the evidence must be easily displayed and explained to jurors in simple terms that people of average intelligence and education can understand. Jurors have a tendency to ignore or give little weight to evidence they do not understand. This is a major complication with DNA evidence. The nature of the science is complex and confusing, making visual displays and strong statistics very important to the use of DNA as evidence.

ODDS, CALCULATIONS, AND STATISTICS

The statistics in table 2 are based on calculations made using a formula developed by two scientists, G. H. Hardy and W. Weinberg, in 1908. The Hardy-Weinberg Principle, as their discovery came to be known, can be used to calculate how common any *allele* (different forms of a gene) may be in a population based on some simple principles of genetics.

Every person in the world has two copies of every gene in their genome. One is inherited from her father, the other from her mother. Some common alleles include those for hair color or eye color. The color of a person's hair is controlled by the combination of alleles for the hair color gene that they inherited from their parents.

Sometimes, the genes are identical, even though they have come from two different sources. When the two genes are identical, we say that the person is *homozygous* for that particular gene. A person having two different alleles for a gene is said to be *heterozygous* for that gene. Alleles can also be *dominant* or *recessive*. Using the frequency of the recessive allele, which can be determined by examining an individual's family tree, a

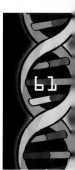

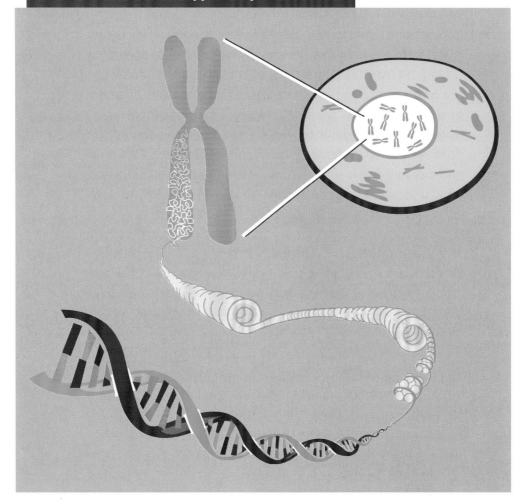

Genetic information is carried on the chromosomes; therefore, through the generations, half is inherited from the mother and half from the father.

scientist can calculate the odds of inheriting the different alleles of that gene. Once the allele frequencies are known, scientists can easily figure out the odds of any one person having a certain pattern of alleles. The calculation is relatively simple once the frequencies are known.

To calculate the frequency of any two people having the same profile as shown in table 2, visit http://www.csfs.ca/

pplus/profiler.htm, the Royal Canadian Mounted Police online STR profile calculator. Simply enter the genotype data from table 2 in the proper field and click "calculate." You might notice that there are different databases you can select from before you run your calculation. This is because the frequency of the different STRs varies between ethnic groups. This provides yet another way that DNA profiling accuracy can be increased.

Generally, STR data is reported in table form, as seen on page 57, because that is a nice way to show a jury the number of repeats without confusing them with numbers. Sometimes, though, the actual data is shown. Typically, the STR locus, such as D18S51, is listed first. This is often followed by the genotype, or a listing of which alleles of that locus are present. Look at table 2 and you will see that for D18S51, the alleles are 12 and 13. This means that the individual is heterozygous for D18S51, and there are twelve repeats in one allele, and thirteen repeats in the other. Following the genotype is the frequency of that particular genotype in the population. In other words, for D18S51, 4.3 percent of the population has this particular genotype.

By using all thirteen STRs recommended by the FBI, forensic biologists can reduce the odds that a particular sample of DNA could have come from more than one person to less than one in 3 trillion. It might seem impossible that all this information could be useful to a forensic biologist fighting a crime, or to a prosecutor working to get a guilty verdict. Without a way to quickly and easily check the evidence, it might be. DNA databases, however, are the glue that holds it all together.

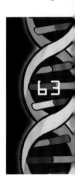

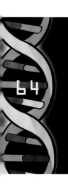

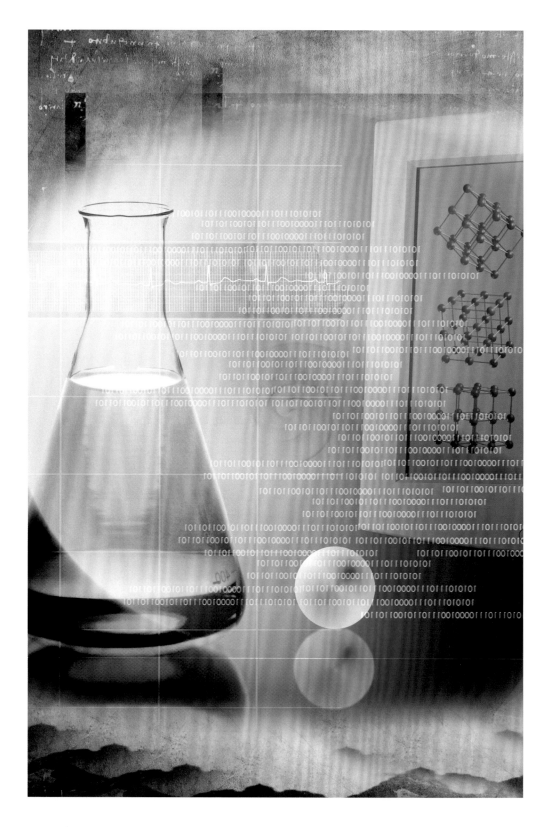

CHAPTER FIVE

The Use of DNA Databases to Catch Criminals

In 1993, a man broke into a young woman's apartment in Cincinnati, Ohio. He woke her up and raped her at knifepoint. The man left plenty of evidence at the scene of the crime, including semen, which contained DNA that could be used for comparison with suspects' DNA. Unfortunately, no suspect could be located that matched the DNA sample, and this horrible crime went unsolved for a number of years.

The young woman would have to wait nearly ten years for a major break in the case. It did not come from a new witness stepping forward or a surprise confession like you might see on a television show. It actually came from a computer.

The State of Ohio instituted a program to take DNA samples from inmates convicted of certain crimes. Those DNA samples are analyzed and placed into a computer database for comparison with samples found at the scene of unsolved crimes. One day, the computer found a match between the DNA of a man serving a sentence for aggravated burglary and the DNA that was found in the semen at the Cincinnati rape.

Rodney J. Crooks had paid his debt to society, serving almost seven years in prison, but the day he was released was

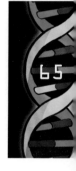

also the day he was *indicted* for another crime. Although he attempted to defend himself against these charges, he couldn't explain the presence of his semen inside the rape victim. He did claim they had *consensual* intercourse, but he could not provide evidence of any relationship with the young woman whatsoever, and his story did not convince many. The judge in the case, Judge Robert Reuhlman, said, "You gave this ridiculous story that it was some love affair, something like that. . . . You broke into her apartment, woke her up, raped her, cut her. To use a defense like that is a slap in the face to society and the victim." Without the use of the computer database, Rodney Crooks might still be roaming the streets.

COMPUTER DATABASES: CHANGING THE FACE OF FORENSIC SCIENCE

As DNA profiling has grown, forensic scientists have discovered many ways that the technology can be used to catch criminals. One of the most important recent developments has been the use of computerized databases to share DNA profile information between law enforcement agencies. DNA samples recovered from all manner of crimes can be quickly and easily checked against samples gathered by other states or the FBI to find out if the criminal's identity is known, and if he has committed crimes in other states.

All fifty states now have regulations in place requiring that DNA samples be collected from all convicted offenders and submitted to the federal database, the Combined DNA Index System (CODIS). Investigators who have not been able to identify a suspect in a crime can now search the database in hopes that the criminal has left DNA evidence at other crime scenes or is already in jail for a previous offense. The ability to catalog and search such a collection of DNA evidence allows investigators to solve crimes that might otherwise go unsolved. The value of this capability is obvious: crimes committed by repeat

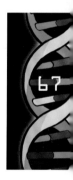

The advent of computer databases allows DNA evidence to be useful to law enforcement in not only confirming whether a known suspect committed a crime, but in actually identifying suspects. Until the creation of such databases, DNA evidence was mostly used to match a sample found at the scene of a crime with that of an already identified suspect. However, some experts believe that in the future, DNA evidence will help forensic scientists early in the investigation process in a whole new way. It may be able to provide much more information that will help the police identify suspects, even ones who are not in any database. The Human Genome Project, a scientific project that mapped out the DNA in humans, has helped us identify what specific areas of DNA relate to particular traits. For example, scientists can now tell by looking at a strand of DNA whether or not the person that it belonged to has red hair. As science progresses, we may be able to gather more information about a person simply by looking at her DNA, which can then help police identify suspects.

offenders will be far easier to solve due to the ability to easily identify suspects.

CODIS is actually a three-tiered system, relying on input from local, state, and national databases. Local crime labs send

CODIS links the information collected by different law enforcement agencies, making new information available to each of them.

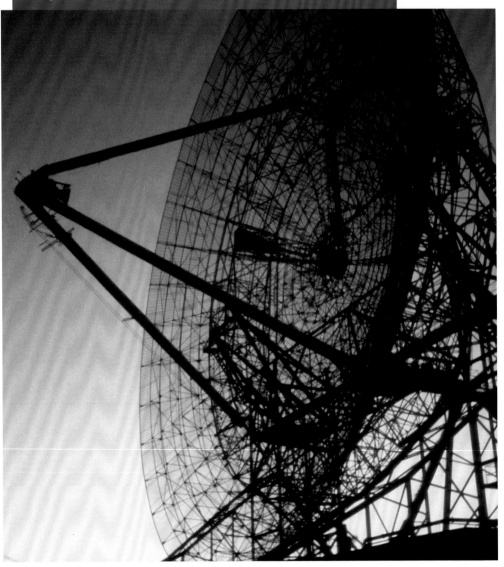

their data to a state database. State databases are then linked to the National DNA Index System (NDIS). Because of differences in state laws and regulations, each state maintains control over the DNA evidence it submits. The combination of all three tiers is what we know as CODIS.

Even in its early testing stages, the CODIS database proved to be invaluable for law enforcement. In 1993, when the software was first released to a selection of forensic laboratories around the country, Minnesota investigators became the first in the nation to identify a suspect based on a DNA match. At the time, Minnesota had a state DNA database containing 1,200 profiles. Crime laboratory technicians matched DNA evidence found at the scene of a rape and murder with that of a convicted felon already in the state database, positively identifying the attacker. When confronted with the evidence, the man quickly admitted to the crimes, indicating that the database could be successful on a national scale. Imagine the excitement in law enforcement circles!

In a similar case, police in Miami were able to link an unsolved 1991 rape case to a man serving a sentence for a sexual assault committed in Orlando in 1993. The convicted man had committed a crime in Miami and moved to Orlando to escape the pressure of the police investigation. His second crime, however, is typical of many offenders, a fact that makes the CODIS database so useful: many criminals do not commit one crime and then stop. Repeat offenders often move about the country to avoid being caught, making the use of a database like CODIS vital in tracking their movements.

There are many more stories of law enforcement officers around the country using the database to match the suspect in one crime with the convicted criminal of another. Every state has reported success in solving crimes that would otherwise have been tough to crack, saving thousands of dollars and probably many lives in the process. Getting criminals off the streets is a great way to ensure that people of your town live safer lives.

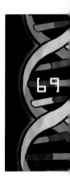

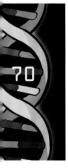

The CODIS database contains over 1.6 million DNA profiles, and the number grows by thousands every year. The majority of the samples come from convicted criminals, but the number of samples taken from families of missing persons and from the scenes of unsolved crimes continues to grow. An unfortunate side effect of the success of the CODIS database is that, as more and more cases are cataloged, the search times for evidence grows as well. At present, many state crime labs have a backlog because they do not have enough manpower to keep up with the number of DNA profiles that need to be developed each day. Most states have increased funding to full-service crime laboratories so that more forensic biologists can be hired to handle the overwhelming amount of data. Although computers get faster and smarter every year, it can still be very time consuming for even the best computers to sort through the huge number of profiles on the computer while searching for a match.

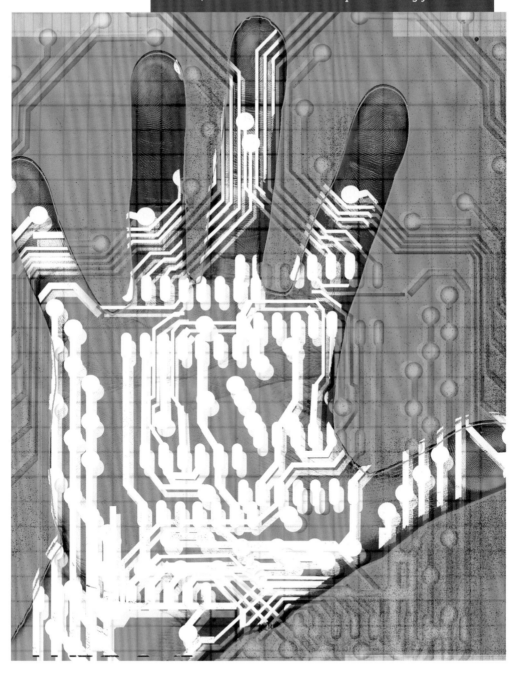

The CODIS database helps in comparing the genetic information of unknown remains to the families of missing loved ones, and can be a valuable step in reuniting families.

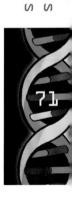

Criminal cases are not the only way the CODIS database has been a success. Around the country, thousands of missing persons are reported each year. Families that are desperate for answers have found that the database is a good way to help track down their missing loved ones. DNA from relatives has been used to find runaways and to identify unknown remains found in remote locations.

In 2004, CODIS technicians reported that 10,000 "hits" had been recorded by the system. This means that around the country, 10,000 DNA profiles from unknown sources had been positively matched with a profile recorded in the database. Those are some pretty good numbers! Another indicator of the success of CODIS in the United States is that other nations are developing their own DNA databases. As they say, imitation is the greatest form of flattery. At present, CODIS is not connected to any other databases in the world, but this may change. Imagine being able to share forensic information around the globe. Committing a crime and fleeing the country would be less attractive then!

ETHICAL CONCERNS: THE GATTACA CONCEPT

In the 1997 movie *Gattaca*, which starred Ethan Hawke and Uma Thurman, DNA information contained in national databases was used to discriminate against people based on their genetic makeup. In this fictional portrayal, a person's DNA profile determined what school he would go to and what jobs he could get. A person whose DNA had been engineered for high intelligence would go to the best schools and get appealing jobs, while a person whose DNA indicated low levels of intelligence would be trained for menial jobs.

While this may seem far-fetched, this very risk is a source of worry for some people. Many individuals see an ethical problem with entering highly personal information, such as a DNA profile, into a national database. The primary concern is that

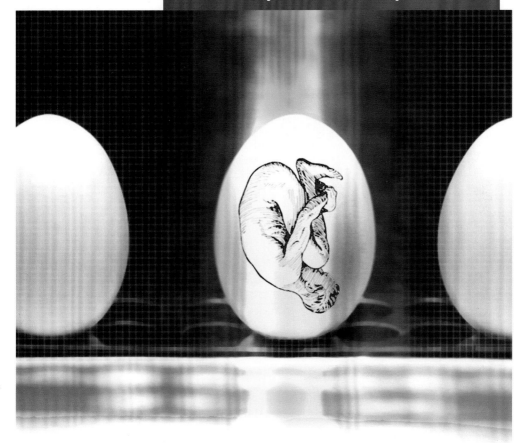

Critics of the CODIS database argue that the collection of an individual's genetic information is an invasion of privacy that may have dire social consequences.

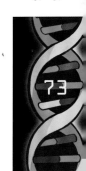

doing so would be an invasion of privacy, moving us closer to the situation in the movie. The main point made by opponents of the CODIS database is that insurance companies, employers, and others could use the information improperly. While these are valid concerns, in fact, the CODIS database does not contain any information about the actual genes a person may have

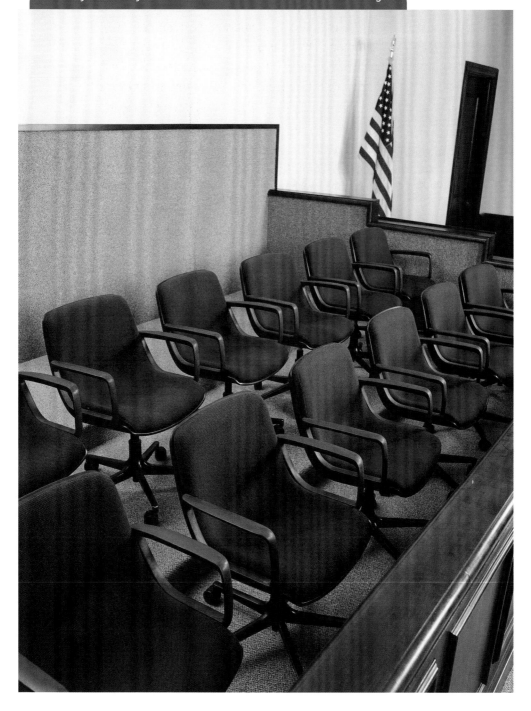

The information found in DNA can be crucial in a court setting.

in their genome. Rather, a DNA profile has thirteen tiny snap-shots of very small regions of a person's DNA. This information cannot tell an insurance company whether an individual will get cancer or what traits that person will exhibit. In addition, the general public will not be cataloged in the system. It would be almost impossible for CODIS to handle DNA profiles for every citizen of the United States. The time and effort required by such a project would easily prevent anyone from trying to take it on.

Some advocates have argued that criminals' rights are being ignored when DNA samples are taken after a conviction. Convicted criminals, they say, remain citizens and therefore should retain the protections given to citizens. But is entering a DNA profile into a database truly an invasion of privacy? Is it all that different from a company keeping logs of the credit card numbers of people who have made purchases at their company?

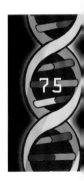

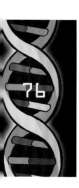

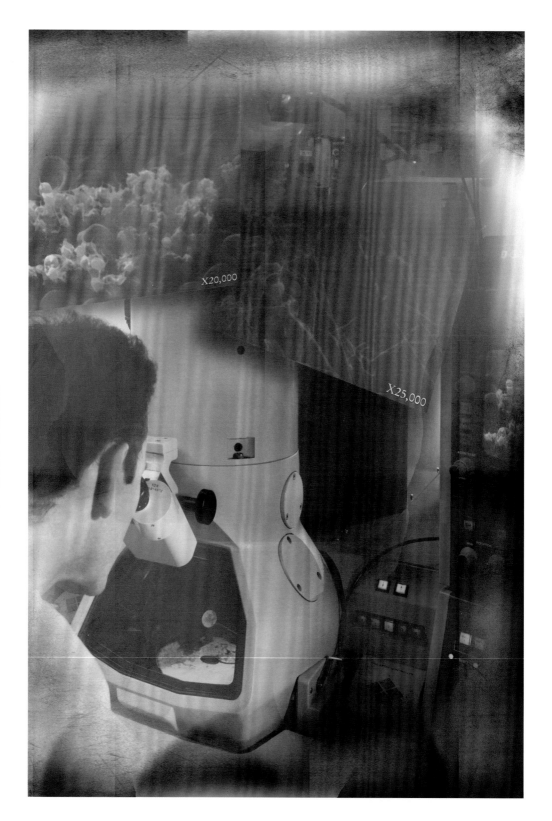

CHAPTER SIX

Tools of the Trade

On September 7, 1981, Yvonne Fine was found strangled to death in her New Hampshire home. Examination of her remains revealed she had been sexually assaulted prior to her death. Shortly after the discovery of the crime, a suspect was arrested. Yvonne's clothing had a useable amount of semen on it and was stored in a freezer as evidence. A man named Joseph Whittey was soon convicted of rape and murder for the crime.

In 1999, as a part of the state's DNA database effort, the samples from Yvonne's clothing were used to develop a DNA profile for Whittey. The clothing was sent to Cellmark laboratories, the same company that provided the expert witness for the prosecution in the O. J. Simpson trial. The samples were gathered from the clothing and DNA successfully extracted. The samples were then PCR amplified with the thirteen core loci according to FBI guidelines, using the standard kit and DNA analysis equipment. Cellmark expert, Dr. Robin Cotton, processed the evidence and concluded that the DNA from the semen sample matched Joseph Whittey.

In 2003, Whittey appealed the conviction, claiming a host of errors from the original trial. As a result, the state attorney

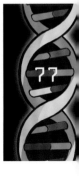

78

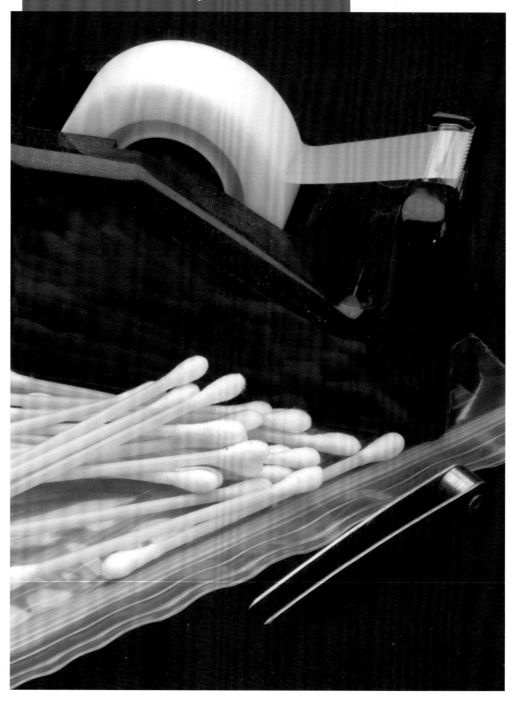

Low-tech but vital forensic tools

general ordered all evidence reexamined. Whittey and his attorney filed several motions in an effort to get his original conviction thrown out and to make the new DNA evidence inadmissible. The argument was that Cellmark had not used equipment and kits that met the requirements set forth by the courts in a previous case. The attorney argued that the STR equipment was not sensitive or accurate enough to be admitted in court.

Unfortunately for Whittey, by the time his case was heard by a court of appeals, the number of cases in which STR evidence had been used had grown to a very large number. DNA databases were also growing rapidly, and the federal government had thrown its weight behind getting all states to collect DNA samples from all convicted felons. It soon became clear that the equipment was in fact very accurate, having been used for thousands of DNA profiles. The occurrence of errors had been very low and was decreasing steadily as the system was refined. Since the thirteen STRs used by Cellmark for the identification were the same ones recommended by the FBI, the judges ruled Whittey's appeal had no basis. Joseph Whittey remains in prison.

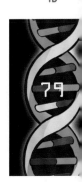

EQUIPMENT FOR GATHERING EVIDENCE

As with any high-tech work, DNA profiling uses a number of very specialized (and very expensive) pieces of equipment—but the entire process starts with a few low-tech, very cheap tools: a cotton swab, some sticky tape, tweezers, and a plastic or paper bag.

At most crime scenes, a huge amount of unseen evidence is available to be gathered by the trained crime-scene investigator. If she finds some sort of fluid, she must carefully collect a sample with a cotton swab. If hairs are visible, tweezers can be used to pick them up and place them in evidence bags. Where there are carpets or other places hairs might hide, sticky tape can be used to lift fibers that might provide clues. New

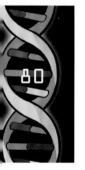

The National Institute of Justice, an agency that is part of the U.S. Department of Justice, has put out a checklist of items that should be collected by crime-scene investigators when looking for DNA evidence. The recommended items include fingernail clippings, tissues, paper towels, napkins, cotton swabs, toothpicks, cigarette butts, straws, and anything else that has come into contact with the mouth, bedding, dirty laundry, hats, eyeglasses or contact lenses, used envelopes or stamps, used condoms, or bullets that have passed through bodies. None of these items require high-tech equipment for collection.

techniques have even been developed to collect skin cells from doorknobs the perpetrator might have touched. These cells can be a valuable source of DNA, and the simple cotton swab is the tool of choice for collecting them.

A crime-scene investigator may use a slightly more high-tech piece of equipment, such as a UV light source, in order to locate semen that might yield DNA evidence. Anyone who has watched an episode or two of *CSI* has seen the investigators

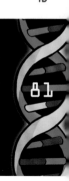

However menial it may seem to our everyday lives, the cotton swab is an important component of the forensic scientist's tool kit.

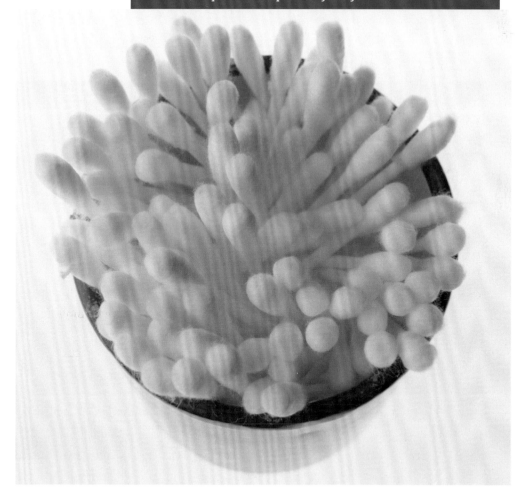

turn out the lights, turn on an ALS (alternate light source), and watch stains glow. Although it is not always as simple in real life as it is on television, semen will *fluoresce* quite quickly under UV light. This can provide the investigator with an indication of what areas should be swabbed for DNA evidence.

EQUIPMENT FOR ANALYZING DNA

Once the evidence is collected, it is brought to the forensic laboratory for analysis. Here, the various forensic scientists begin their work, trying to find useful information from the pieces of evidence provided to them by the crime-scene investigators.

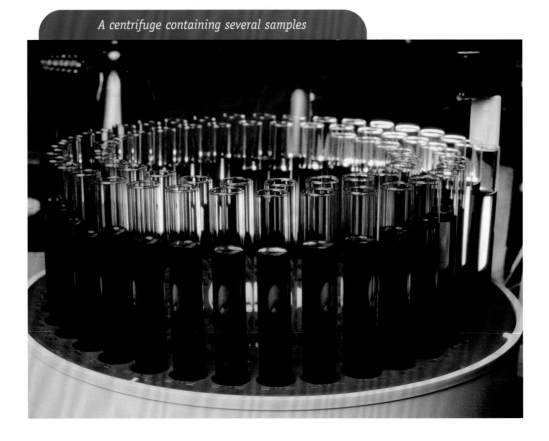
A centrifuge containing several samples

The forensic biologist gathers the evidence that might contain DNA and goes to work, using the many critical pieces of equipment in a forensic biology laboratory.

The first step of any DNA analysis is the extraction process. For this, the biologist uses special chemicals that break down the cells but leave the DNA intact. A hot water bath, a small tub that keeps the water at the right temperature, is usually used to run the extraction reaction. This tool is necessary because cells are less stable and easier to break down at higher temperatures, making the job the chemicals have to do easier. Once the cells are broken down, a machine called a centrifuge is used to remove all the pieces of the cells, so they don't interfere with later reactions.

Centrifuges in forensic laboratories used to be large (dishwasher sized or larger) machines that needed much space. Not so anymore! Most centrifuges are now smaller than the monitor of a typical computer, and they sit on laboratory bench tops. The samples a forensic biologist works with are usually very small and can be centrifuged effectively in the smaller machines. Centrifuges have a circular rack with holes designed to hold standard-sized tubes used most often for PCR. The machine has a powerful electric motor that can spin the rack around at more than 12,000 rotations per minute (RPM). When the tubes holding a sample are centrifuged, the cell fragments in the extraction solution are separated by density. The densest parts, like the cell membrane, are forced to the bottom of the tube, where they form a pellet. The fluid remaining in the tube contains the DNA and some proteins. This is poured into a new tube, which is centrifuged again for a longer period of time to remove the proteins and any remaining cell parts from the fluid. The DNA remains in the fluid, which can be used directly in the PCR amplification. In the event that the scientist will not have time to finish the entire process, the sample can be frozen once the proteins are all removed from the fluid.

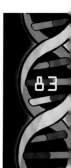

84

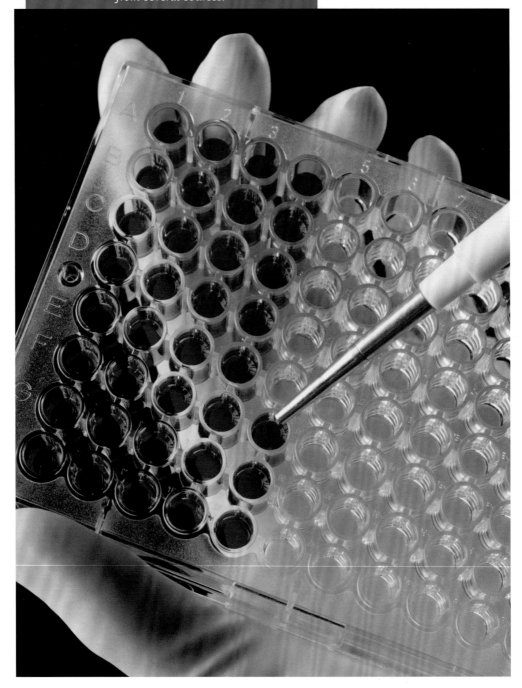

Scientists can extract and analyze DNA samples from several sources.

Forensic laboratories have specialized freezers that can accurately keep the temperature of –112 degrees Fahrenheit (–80 degrees Celsius). This extremely cold temperature is important for storing DNA for a very long time. Part of the job of a forensic scientist is to keep samples of the evidence, just in case they are needed later. Many *cold cases* have been reopened and solved years later when new technologies became available to examine the evidence.

Typically, once the DNA is extracted, the forensic biologist must find out just how much DNA she was able to recover from the cells. A UV spectrophotometer is used to determine the amount of DNA in a sample. UV spectrophotometers fire a beam of light through the sample, allowing the biologist to calculate with remarkable accuracy how much DNA is in the tube. Most molecules will react with light if it is the correct wavelength, absorbing some of the energy in the light beam. DNA absorbs light in the UV spectrum at a wavelength of 260 *nanometers*. The light beam passes through the sample to a lens on the other side of the sample vial, and the computer inside the spectrophotometer determines how much light was absorbed. A more concentrated DNA sample absorbs more light than a less-concentrated one. The biologist uses a mathematical formula to figure out the amount of DNA by using the number provided by the machine.

Once the amount of DNA is calculated, the sample can be broken down into smaller tubes so some can be saved. The biologist takes one of the smaller tubes and combines the DNA sample with a set of chemicals required for the thermocycler, which the forensic biologist can use to change the temperature of a sample very quickly through a range of different temperatures. Some have four different aluminum blocks, each set at a different temperature, and a computerized arm that moves the samples from one block to the next as the cycles progress. Others have just one block and special heating and cooling elements that can change temperature very rapidly. Each stage of a PCR cycle requires very specific temperatures, and the

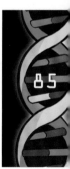

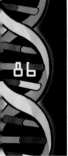

The thermocycler is a tool that makes the work of forensic biologists much easier by automating the heating and cooling necessary for PCR. This machine was developed based on the work of the Nobel Prize–winning scientist, Kary B. Mullis, the creator of the PCR method. Unlike today's scientists, who can simply place a DNA sample into a thermocycler with the proper chemicals and come back a couple hours later to millions of copies of DNA, Mullis had to do all of the heating and cooling himself. He used the relatively low-tech tools of hot water and ice water baths to repeatedly change the temperature of the mixture, eventually figuring out what temperatures for which lengths of time worked best for the process.

thermocycler makes the rapid change of temperature possible. Before the development of this machine, scientists had to set up water baths at each temperature and move the samples by hand from bath to bath, often taking as long as three hours. The benefits of the thermocycler in this case are obvious.

Once the DNA samples are amplified, the real examination can begin. The samples are injected into a machine called a capillary electrophoresis DNA analyzer. This machine is large, often filling a space the size of a refrigerator. It is mostly automated, allowing the forensic biologist the freedom to place the samples to be analyzed in it and go work on something else. Most often, these machines have special containers that

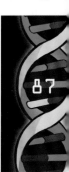

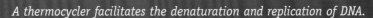

A thermocycler facilitates the denaturation and replication of DNA.

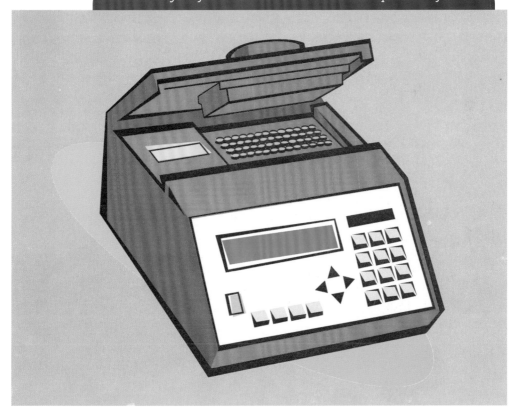

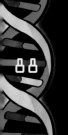

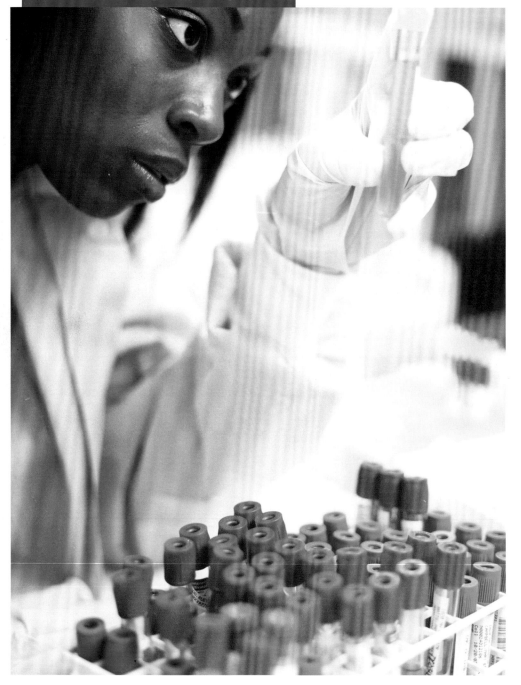

The centrifuge allows scientists to separate DNA from other parts of a sample.

will hold as many as ninety-six different samples. Once the samples have been placed in the sample tray, a special needle on a computerized arm is inserted into each sample, one at a time, and a small amount of sample is drawn up into the machine. The sample is moved through the machine as an electrical current forces the DNA from one end of a tiny tube to the other. In much the same fashion as a UV spectrophotometer, light at a certain wavelength is passed through the tube, and the DNA reacts with the light. The computerized brain of the DNA analyzer can interpret the results of the reactions and output a graph that shows how many repeats of each STR are in the sample. The number of repeats determines a person's DNA profile.

Obviously, this is a complicated procedure. You may think it all sounds so confusing that you'd never want to consider a career in forensic biology. But if you like science, you may find that combining biology and crime-solving is a career you want to consider.

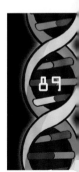

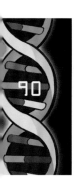

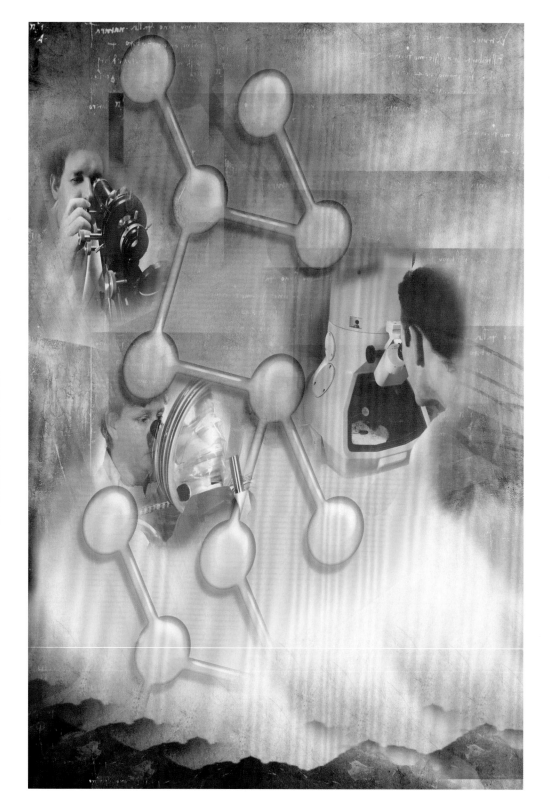

CHAPTER SEVEN

Forensic Biology:
A Promising Career?

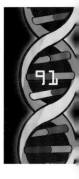

In the world of forensic science, few people are as well known as Dr. Henry Lee. He has been involved in over six thousand cases around the world, including the Jon Benet Ramsey case, Bosnian and Croatian war crimes cases, a review of the President John Kennedy assassination case, and the suicide of President Clinton's White House attorney, Vince Foster. Lee served as an expert defense witness in the O. J. Simpson trial. There are hundreds of cases in which Dr. Lee has served as a consultant or expert witness.

Dr. Lee's education began with a degree in police science from the Central Police College of Taiwan. He went on to serve as captain of the Taipei police force in Taiwan, and after ten years as chief, he came to the United States, where he studied forensic science at John Jay College of Criminal Justice. With a bachelor of science degree in forensic science in hand, he went on to New York University and completed a master of science degree, as well as a Ph.D. in biochemistry.

In 1975, after completing his doctoral studies, Dr. Lee was hired as the first professor of forensic science at New Haven

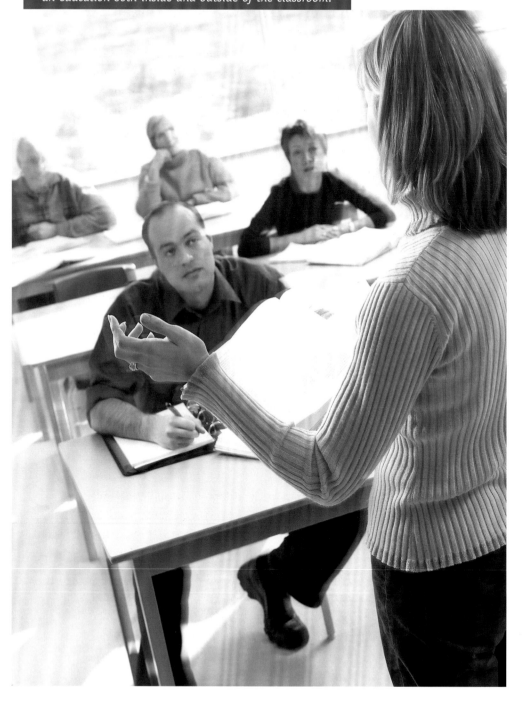

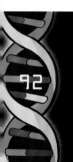
Preparing for a career in the forensic sciences requires an education both inside and outside of the classroom.

University in Connecticut. He remained on the faculty there until 1979, when he took a position as Connecticut's chief criminalist, helping to build the police force into one of the most modern units in the country.

Dr. Lee's experience and education made him a prime candidate for writing textbooks and journal articles about many areas of forensic science, especially the biological and physical sciences. He is among the most honored members in the U.S. forensic science community, having earned several honorary doctoral degrees and various awards from the American Academy of Forensic Sciences. Dr. Lee has been one of the models for a new age of forensic scientists, eager to be successful in their chosen careers in crime fighting.

MEET YOUR FORENSIC BIOLOGIST

Operating the equipment in a forensic biology laboratory is not just a matter of following instructions. The skills needed to take a small sample of DNA and make it useful take a long time to cultivate. Practice is the key because forensic biologists often work with tiny amounts of materials, invisible even under a microscope. A small mistake while handling the evidence can mean the difference between a conviction and an acquittal. Proper training is therefore very important for the prospective forensic molecular biologist.

All forensic scientists are required to meet very strict training requirements, because the evidence and cases they handle have the potential to change—or even end—a person's life. Making mistakes is simply not acceptable. Forensic biologists must go through several years of college. The requirements vary from state to state, but all require at least a bachelor of science degree from an accredited college. People wishing to work in this technologically advanced field often have completed a master of science or even a doctoral program.

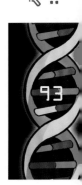

DEGREE PATH TO A CAREER IN A FORENSIC BIOLOGY LABORATORY

The requirements for a person wishing to work as a forensic biologist are dependent on state regulations for the position, and they vary from state to state and province to province. In all states, however, a person wishing to enter a career in a forensic molecular laboratory must first complete at least a bachelor

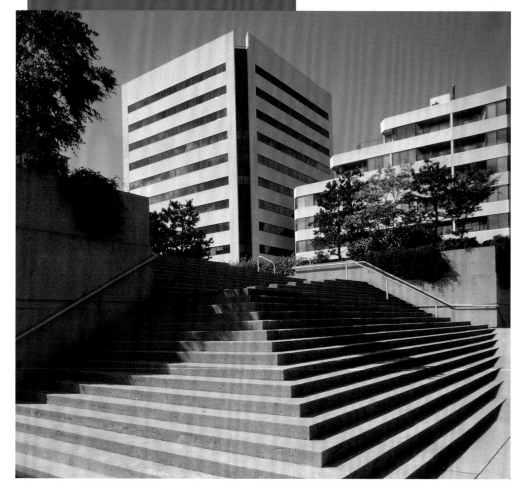

Before becoming a forensic biologist, you must go through several years of college.

Over the last ten years, the number of colleges and universities offering programs specifically designed to prepare students for careers in forensic science has skyrocketed. Literally hundreds of universities in the United States and around the world offer forensic science programs. These colleges offer a wide variety of programs, from associate's degrees all the way up through doctorates. Some have a specific focus, such as Lock Haven University's concentration in Forensic DNA, while others are just general forensic science programs. The American Academy of Forensic Sciences maintains a list of these colleges on its Web site at www.aafs.org/default.asp?section_id=resources&page_id=colleges_and_universities#UNDERGRADUATE%20PROGRAMS.

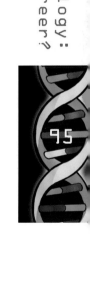

of science degree in some related field. Commonly, individuals working in forensic biology laboratories hold degrees in forensic science or biology, with a focus on molecular biology, genetics, or biochemistry, in accordance with FBI recommendations. The courses typical of college science programs are designed to provide a good basis of information, but they are very general. A student wishing to become a forensic biologist needs to have a good plan as to which courses to take. Four years of college can easily be filled with general science classes that do little to actually prepare a person for a demanding career in forensic science.

Perhaps the most effective way to learn about the ins and outs of working in a forensic biology laboratory is to get an internship. Being inside the laboratory day in and day out is a great way to get valuable experience and to make sure that forensic biology is the right career track for you. Most of the time, interns do the little tasks that need to get done, such as washing glassware or cleaning the benches, but being around the scientists as they do their work lets students see how things really work in the laboratory. The majority of interns come away from their time in the laboratory with an increased understanding and appreciation for the job. Internships should be done as early in a student's academic career as possible to allow time for changes of heart and career paths, just in case. In addition, students often learn they will want to take certain courses so they can improve their understanding of aspects of the job they might have found particularly challenging.

In general, most students wishing to work as forensic biologists will want to take certain courses to advance their knowledge in the areas of science on which crime-solving relies heavily on a daily basis. Forensic biologists are often called on to testify in the cases they have worked on, so a firm understanding of genetics is critical. When called on in a court case, a forensic biologist must be able to describe clearly what the evidence indicates. Jurors must understand the basics of genetics before they will accept DNA evidence and give it equal weight

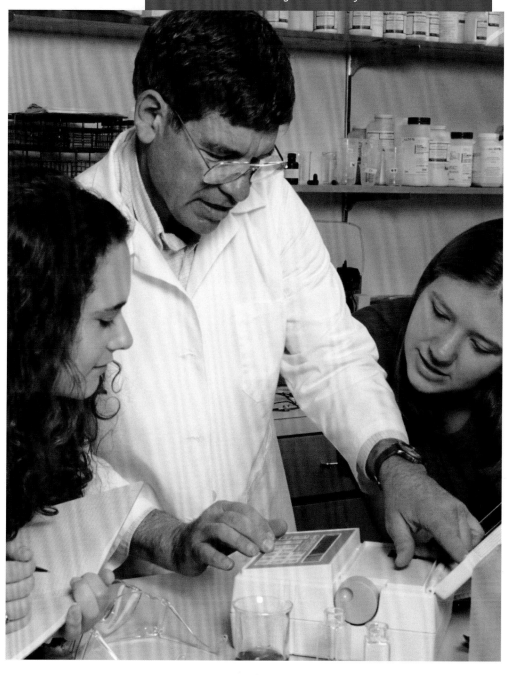

Interns sometimes have to do the little tasks that need to be done, but their time spent in the lab may prove invaluable when considering a career in forensic science.

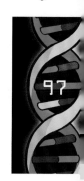

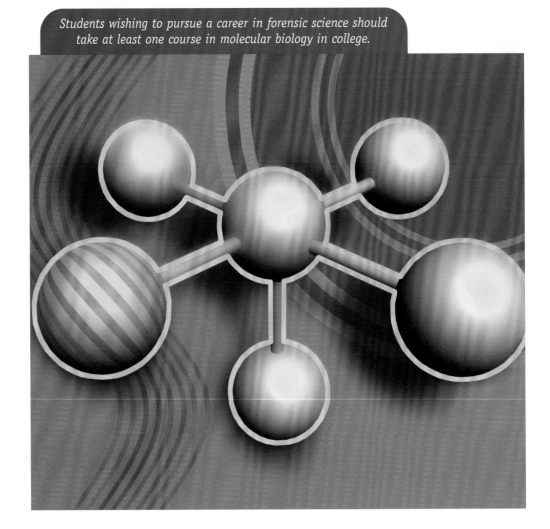

in a trial. A forensic biologist who has a firm understanding of the theories of genetics will be far more able to explain them to jurors.

Molecular biology courses are an important part of understanding how the DNA profiling process works and why. Most colleges with a biology curriculum offer at least one course in molecular biology, where students are taught about the structure and form of DNA. These courses give an individual a sound

Students wishing to pursue a career in forensic science should take at least one course in molecular biology in college.

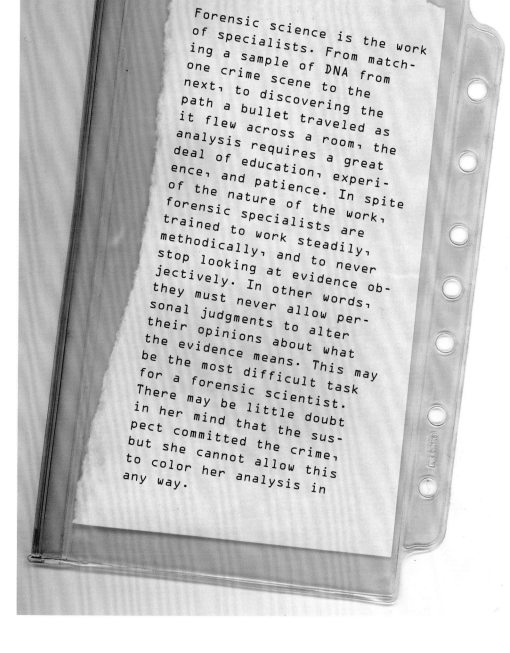

Forensic science is the work of specialists. From matching a sample of DNA from one crime scene to the next, to discovering the path a bullet traveled as it flew across a room, the analysis requires a great deal of education, experience, and patience. In spite of the nature of the work, forensic specialists are trained to work steadily, methodically, and to never stop looking at evidence objectively. In other words, they must never allow personal judgments to alter their opinions about what the evidence means. This may be the most difficult task for a forensic scientist. There may be little doubt in her mind that the suspect committed the crime, but she cannot allow this to color her analysis in any way.

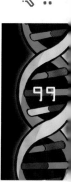

basis to understand how and why the PCR process works. A forensic biologist should be able to troubleshoot the procedures, in case the standard methodology does not work for some reason. In addition, understanding the structure of DNA will help the biologist to determine whether an error will have a significant effect on the results, a very important factor in determining whether evidence is acceptable for use in court.

Biochemistry, the study of the chemical behavior of biological molecules, helps a forensic biologist understand the effect of different chemicals on the reactions they use, and whether any contaminant from the surrounding environment could ruin their results.

Each of the science courses mentioned above is likely to have a laboratory requirement along with the normal class section. Because forensic biology relies heavily on the use of highly advanced equipment, it is very important for a student pursuing a career in forensics to make the most of the laboratory time. It serves as a great introduction to using many of the tools of the trade, and at some colleges, students will actually have access to every piece of equipment used in a forensic biology laboratory.

Statistics courses help forensic biologists understand the results of their work in the laboratory. Their job involves explaining their findings to others, particularly jurors. A forensic scientist who assumes people will understand the meanings of the statistics behind the use of STRs as evidence is asking for trouble in court. He must be able to speak clearly and accurately about what the results mean in order to encourage the jury to pay attention to his findings.

Some colleges offer forensic science courses as electives or as part of a forensic science focus. These courses are not prerequisites for a career as a forensic biologist, but they may increase a student's understanding of the theories and practices used in law enforcement and forensics in general. In addition, forensic biologists often find useful coursework in law, courtroom procedures, and public speaking.

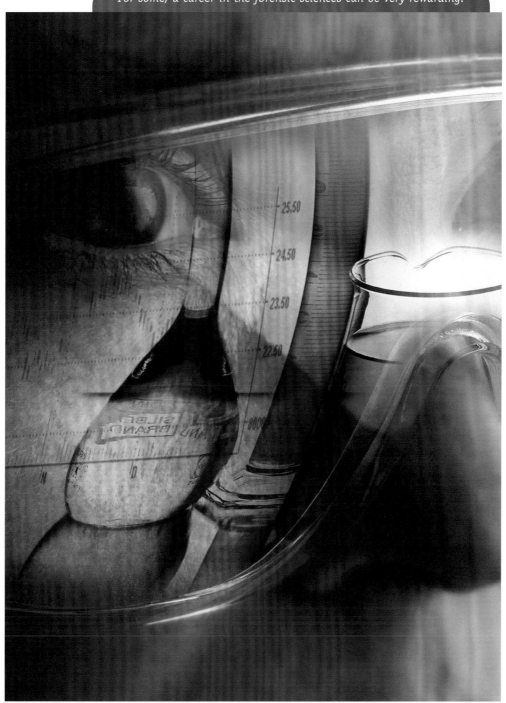

For some, a career in the forensic sciences can be very rewarding.

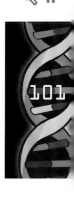

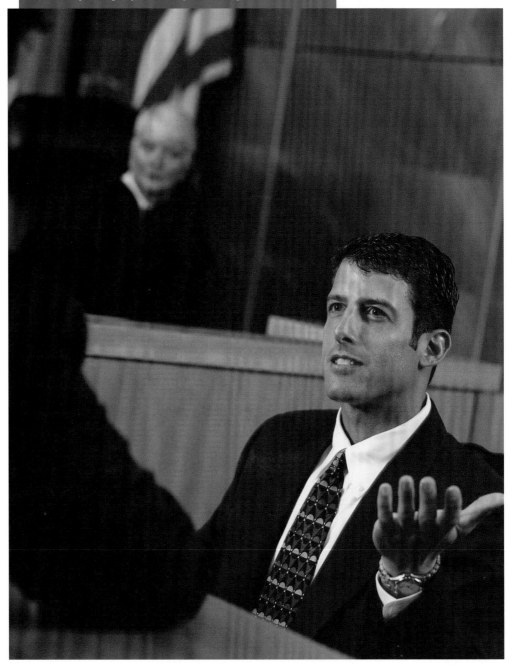

Forensic scientists are sometimes called into court as expert witnesses to explain the complicated findings of a scientific investigation.

Students who can work on an independent research project in genetics or molecular biology may have an advantage over others in that they will have more opportunities to use the equipment, and develop more confidence in their ability to do so properly. Many students graduate from four-year colleges having never actually performed a true experiment. An independent study project can change that. Independent studies, if done properly, will serve as an introduction to the use of forensic equipment, troubleshooting when there are problems, interpreting results, and reporting findings. Forensic biologists do these things on a regular, if not daily basis. Practice makes perfect, as they say, and it is the only real way to become proficient with the equipment used in a forensic laboratory. Only those who truly master the equipment and techniques will become experts in their field.

EXPERT TESTIMONY

Once the science is done and the evidence examined, forensic scientists often have one major additional job: to present that evidence in a criminal court. Expert testimony is a part of many court cases. Some experts testify as part of their jobs, such as medical examiners or other government employees. Other independent experts are paid a handsome fee to analyze the evidence and appear in court, often presenting an alternative view of the evidence than that which was given by the other witnesses.

In order to testify in court, experts must be qualified, meaning that the expert must establish his credentials and training in front of the jury. He should expect to answer questions relating to articles or books he has published, his schooling, his area of expertise, positions he has held, and anything else that adds or takes away from his *credibility* as an expert. Judges can refuse to qualify an expert if his expertise is not established.

Once an expert is qualified, she gets extra leeway with her testimony. Most witnesses are limited to answering the

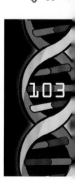

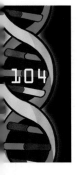

questions asked by attorneys, but experts are allowed to present information to the judge and jury in a much less-structured format, essentially acting as teachers. The testimony they give would often be far too technical and confusing if they were not given the opportunity to explain it in detail.

Being a forensic biologist is not an easy job. The daily routine can become boring and dull at times, but the rewards are potentially great. Few people in the world can actually say they helped put a dangerous criminal behind bars, especially on a daily basis, or that they helped find someone's missing loved one. Forensic biologists have important jobs, but they often find themselves working silently in the background, doing their part to make the world safer for us all.

Glossary

allele: One of two or more alternative forms of a gene, occupying the same position on paired chromosomes and controlling the same inherited trait.

amplify: Make larger, greater, or stronger.

anneal: To become tougher, less fragile.

buffer: Solution that is able to maintain a constant ph, even when acids or bases are added to it.

cold cases: Crimes that have not been solved but are no longer being actively investigated.

consensual: Involving the agreement of all involved.

credibility: The ability to inspire trust and belief.

dominant: More important, effective, or prominent than others.

error rate: The number of defective steps in a transaction.

extension: A piece that has been added to make something longer.

fluoresce: To emit light when exposed to radiation or bombarding particles.

geneticists: People who study or are experts in genetic heredity.

genome: The complete genetic information an individual organism inherits from its parents.

heterozygous: A term used to describe a cell or organism that has two or more different versions of at least one of its genes.

homozygous: Having two identical genes at the corresponding loci of homologous chromosomes.

indicted: To charge someone formally with a crime.

loci: The positions of genes in a chromosome.

mitochondrion: A small round or rod-shaped body found in cytoplasm of most cells and that produces enzymes used for metabolism.

molecular biologists: Scientists who study the nature and function of biological phenomena at their molecular levels.

nanometers: Billionths of a meter.

organelles: Specialized parts of a cell that have their own functions.

peer review: Assessment of an article, piece of work, or research by people who are experts on the subject.

primers: A molecular substrate (substance upon which an enzyme acts) needed in the polymerization reaction that produces another molecule.

prosecution: The party bringing criminal charges.

recanted: Withdrew something previously stated.

recessive: A gene that produces an effect only when its matching allele is identical.

sequenced: Placed in an order.

standardized: Removed variations and irregularities and made all types or examples of something the same or in conformity with one another.

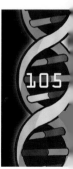

Further Reading

Camenson, Bythe. *Opportunities in Forensic Science Careers*. New York: McGraw-Hill, 2001.

Evans, Colin. *The Casebook of Forensic Detection: How Science Solved 100 of the World's Most Baffling Crimes*. Hoboken, N.J.: Wiley, 1998.

Evans, Colin. *A Question of Evidence: The Casebook of Great Forensic Controversies, From Napoleon to O. J*. Hoboken, N.J.: Wiley, 2002.

Genge, Ngaire. *The Forensic Casebook: The Science of Crime Scene Investigation*. New York: Ballantine Books, 2002.

Lee, Henry C., and Frank Tirnady. *Blood Evidence: How DNA Is Revolutionizing the Way We Solve Crimes*. Cambridge, Mass.: Perseus Publishing, 2002.

Lyle, Douglas P. *Forensics for Dummies*. Hoboken, N.J.: For Dummies, 2004.

Miller, Hugh. *What the Corpse Revealed: Murder and the Science of Forensic Detection*. New York: St. Martin's True Crime Classics, 2000.

Morgan, Marilyn. *Careers in Criminology*. New York: McGraw-Hill, 2000.

Platt, Richard. *Crime Scene: The Ultimate Guide to Forensic Science*. New York: DK Publishing, 2003.

Ramsland, Katherine M. *The Forensic Science of C.S.I.* Berkeley, Calif.: Berkeley Publishing Group, 2001.

Ridley, Matt. *Genome: The Autobiography of a Species in 23 Chapters*. New York: Perennial Publishing, 2000.

Rudin, Norah, and Keith Inman. *An Introduction to Forensic DNA Analysis, 2nd ed*. Boca Raton, Fla.: CRC Press, 2002.

Saferstein, Richard. *Criminalistics: An Introduction to Forensic Science*. Englewood Cliffs, N.J.: Prentice Hall, 2001.

Spencer, Charlotte A. *Genetic Testimony: A Guide to Forensic DNA Profiling*. Englewood Cliffs, N.J.: Prentice Hall, 2003.

For More Information

All About DNA Revolution by Katherine Ramsland
www.crimelibrary.com/criminal_mind/forensics/dna/1.html

An Interview with DNA Forensics Authority Dr. Bruce Weir
www.accessexcellence.org/RC/AB/BA/Interview_Weir.html

Background Information on STRs
www.cstl.nist.gov/biotech/strbase/intro.htm

The Blackett Family DNA Activity—University of Arizona
www.biology.arizona.edu/human_bio/activities/blackett2/overview.html

Can DNA Demand a Verdict?
gslc.genetics.utah.edu/features/forensics

Combined DNA Index System (CODIS) Homepage
www.fbi.gov/hq/lab/codis/index1.htm

DNA Forensics
www.ornl.gov/sci/techresources/Human_Genome/elsi/forensics.shtml

DNA & Forensics
www.karisable.com/crdna1.htm

FAQS Northeastern Association of Forensic Scientists
www.neafs.org/faqs.htm

Forensic Fact File: DNA Profiling
www.nifs.com.au/FactFiles/DNA/what.asp?page=what&title=
DNA%C2%A0Profiling

Forensic Science, Forensics, and Investigation—Crimelibrary.com
www.crimelibrary.com/criminal_mind/forensics

Forensic Serology
faculty.ncwc.edu/toconnor/425/425lect13.htm

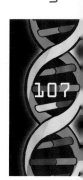

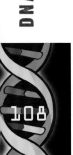

From Fingerprints to DNA—ABC Science Online
www.abc.net.au/science/slab/forensic/default.htm

FBI Handbook of Forensic Science
www.fbi.gov/hq/lab/handbook/intro.htm

Reddy's Forensic Home Page
www.forensicpage.com

Publisher's note:
The Web sites listed on these pages were active at the time of publication.
The publisher is not responsible for Web sites that have changed their addresses or discontinued operation since the date of publication. The publisher will review and update the Web-site list upon each reprint.

Index

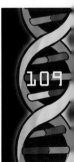

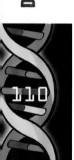

Picture Credits

Artville: pp. 19, 49

Benjamin Stewart: pp. 17, 55, 78

Brand-X: pp. 8, 22, 25, 101

Corbis: pp. 11, 56, 59, 62, 74, 102

Evangeline Ehl: pp. 34, 43, 44, 87

PhotoDisc: pp. 15, 28, 38, 40, 50, 68, 81, 82, 84, 97

Photos.com: pp. 12, 20, 71, 73, 88, 92, 94, 98

To the best knowledge of the publisher, all other images are in the public domain. If any image has been inadvertently uncredited, please notify Harding House Publishing Service, Vestal, New York 13850, so that rectification can be made for future printings.

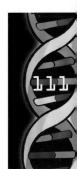

Biographies

AUTHOR

William Hunter lives in Arcade, New York, with his wife, Miranda, and new baby, Elspeth. He is a high school biology and chemistry teacher in upstate New York. He is a graduate of the State University of New York at Buffalo, earning a master's degree in biology. His interest in forensic science led him to complete elective coursework in the forensic science training program at the University of New York at Buffalo. The author has also been involved in the development and testing of a series of forensic science educational activities, as well as a comprehensive activity for a national science conference.

SERIES CONSULTANTS

Carla Miller Noziglia is Senior Forensic Advisor, Tanzania, East Africa, for the U.S. Department of Justice, International Criminal Investigative Training Assistant Program. A Fellow of the American Academy of Forensic Sciences, Ms. Noziglia is Chair of the Board of Trustees of the Forensic Science Foundation since 2001. Her work has earned her many honors and commendations, including Distinguished Fellow from the American Academy of Forensic Sciences (2003) and the Paul L. Kirk Award from the American Academy of Forensic Sciences Criminalistics Section. Ms. Noziglia's publications include *The Real Crime Lab* (coeditor, 2005), *So You Want to be a Forensic Scientist* (coeditor 2003), and contributions to *Drug Facilitated Sexual Assault* (2001), *Convicted by Juries, Exonerated by Science: Case Studies in the Use of DNA* (1996), and the *Journal of Police Science* (1989). She is on the editorial board of the *Journal for Forensic Identification*.

Jay A. Siegel is Director of the Forensic and Investigative Sciences Program in the School of Science at Indiana University, Purdue University, Indianapolis. Dr. Siegel is a Fellow of the American Academy of Forensic Sciences, and is a member of the Forensic Science Society (England) and the editorial board of the *Journal of Forensic Sciences*. His publications include chapters in *Analytical Methods in Forensic Science* (1991), Forensic Science (2002), and *Forensic Science Handbook, vol. 2*. He is the coauthor of the upcoming college textbook *Fundamentals of Forensic Science*. Dr. Siegel has also appeared as an expert witness in many trials and as a forensic expert on television news programs.